I06461608

How to Help Yourself While on Chemotherapy

What Your Body Would Like You To Know

Natalie Mitchell

Cancer Prevention Nutritionist

Copyrighted material

Copyrighted material

The information in this book is based on the experience and research of the author. It is not intended as a substitute for consulting with your physician or other health-care provider. Any attempt to diagnose and treat an illness should be under the direction of a health-care professional. The publisher, author and editor are not responsible for any adverse effects or consequences alleged to result or resulting from the use of any of the suggestions, preparations or procedures discussed in this book.

All rights reserved.

ISBN: 9780988538788

Published by Accretive Solutions Ltd

Mail: PO Box HM 2190, Hamilton HMJX, Bermuda

Editor: Colin Barnes

Cover designer: Craig Laughrey

October 2012

Copyrighted material

Contents

Copyrighted material

"The difference in **winning** *and* **losing** *is most often... **not** **quitting**."*

Walt Disney

Introduction

You are receiving great professional medical treatment from your Doctor and, probably, you feel somewhat distant from participating actively in your fight back to health, which up to now, has been solely in the hands of the medical experts around you. You may suspect, though, that there is actually much you can also do for yourself at this time to help your body overcome your cancer as well as to combat the effect of your chemotherapy treatment. You are so very right!

Your decision to read my book is a powerful affirmation of your motivation and determination to learn how to go about strengthening your body naturally and from within. In my book, I show you, with specific and detailed explanations, how you can greatly enhance your body's natural capability to fight and neutralize the cancer in your body. I will be sharing with you life sustaining information about the kind of nutrition and diet your blood cells are actually craving for to make them even more powerful and effective in defeating active cancer cells in your body. The correct foods and nutrition in your diet at this time will also allow your blood cells and your body to better cope with your chemotherapy treatment's tendency to cause tiredness and fatigue in the body.

I must congratulate you on your decision to read this book which is reflective of your positive attitude about the journey back to health that you are about to begin with your new knowledge and influence in your body's recovery. Nothing is more important in the days and, yes, years ahead as you nurture your body back to being healthy and staying cancer free as a result of what you give your body everyday as fuel to sustain itself in a healthy way.

I thank you for giving me this chance to help you help your body and mind in winning your health back. What you find, in the details within my book, will equip you with the knowledge and methods that I have learned from all around the world over the past 10 years studying with nutritional experts and working with cancer patients. Much of my knowledge of how to strengthen the body to successfully fight cancer I learned from my beloved teacher Marie-France Emele-Ganet, who lives in the Swiss Alps where, for thirty years, she has and continues to successfully treat cancer, diabetic and other patients.

All the knowledge and advice contained in my book is premised on you gaining, as you read, an advanced level of understanding regarding the behavior of our blood cells and what they would ask you to do for them if **they could speak to you right now**. I will talk in more depth on this later in the book but in short, our bodies have very capable defensive mechanisms one of which circulates white blood cells through our bodies to kill sick cells and protect us from other diseases. The body's defensive mechanisms can become weak or damaged just when you need your body to be strongest as you undergo your chemotherapy. My book will teach you how slowly but surely to rebuild and nurture your body's natural defenses to a level where they are doing the very best job in making you healthy and keeping you healthy in the months and years in front of you.

Nutrition, positive thinking, positive emotions and **actions** can deeply influence how susceptible we are to different illnesses. Interestingly, there are many case histories of identical twins where one remains perfectly healthy and the other one develops a serious disease. I see our body as a very intelligent and complex factory created by God and while its complexity does not prevent it sometimes being damaged by cancer cells, it always will respond and do everything it can to cure and **heal itself** provided it is given the necessary environment to do so.

This is where you come in with your new knowledge about what is best for your body at this time. I thank you for allowing me to suggest the paths you should take to optimize the natural healing powers that are already in your body.

In the pages ahead, I encourage you to learn the many, simple yet incredibly powerful, actions you can start taking immediately to create the opportunity for your body to beat your cancer, not just for the short term while you conclude your chemotherapy but for life!

As an illustration of what can be achieved when you want to help your body by taking changes to your nutrition that count, first let me share with you a recent experience with one of my coaching clients. While this story is recent, it is quite unique among many other positive experiences I have seen where patients undergoing chemotherapy are willing to provide their bodies with the types of foods and nutrition that give their blood cells the right fuels they need to have the best chance of overcoming the adverse effects of active cancer cells in their body.

This story began when, I was asked to help a client of mine's friend who we shall call Nigel. This happened after my client became alarmed when he learned his friend Nigel was facing a new cancer issue and about to take a chemotherapy course for the second time in two years.

Nigel was originally diagnosed with bladder cancer two years ago and it was treated successfully with chemotherapy. A few months ago, having had his check at the hospital, doctors found that the cancer had moved to his liver and they recommended to Nigel that he immediately undergo a chemotherapy course again.

As you can imagine, having experienced chemotherapy treatment before, Nigel was not looking forward to another treatment as the earlier course of chemotherapy, while successful, had left Nigel tired, lethargic and with weight loss.

I was subsequently able to appreciate the opportunity to pass on to Nigel much of my knowledge as well as many of the recommendations that are contained in this book, to help him help his body remain strong through the second course of chemotherapy. In addition, I conducted several cancer preventative, immune system strengthening and detoxification coaching sessions with him via Skype. These developments and discussions took place in the couple of months before he started the course. Being a very disciplined and motivated person, Nigel was able to closely follow many of my food and nutritional recommendations, as he, like you, understands that much is within his ability to influence his blood cells to better deal with the cancer cells and the chemotherapy treatment.

Three months later Nigel reported to me that he was benefiting from the nutrition and foods that his body needed, and that chemotherapy was an absolutely more tolerable experience this time compared with his previous course. Throughout the chemotherapy treatment, his energy levels remained high enough that he continued to go to the gym a few times a week and he has been able to continue competitive bicycle racing and running on weekends.

At the halfway point of the current chemotherapy, his Doctors told him the cancer was clearly shrinking and his blood work results were very encouraging.

Now, at the end of his chemotherapy, Doctors have announced that he is FREE of Cancer!

This story is unusual as Nigel was able to create and experience a more satisfactory quality of life with the second chemotherapy course he went through.

Like Nigel, I know you are ready to use your will power, positive attitude and intellect to help your Body, Mind and Spirit conquer your cancer cells and to start feeling better, sustaining your quality of life as you go through your Chemotherapy treatment course.

We shall get down to the details now as you are ready to learn how to immediately Detox your body, start strengthening your immune system and developing more energy while understanding how to move forward to provide and sustain the environment for your body to heal itself now and to stay healthy in the future.

For you to be most successful, it will require your dedication to make some changes to your diet and to continually reinforce your positive attitude to life. With this book, you have everything you need, at your fingertips, to make a difference. It is all in your hands now as you are the caretaker of your precious Mind, Body and Spirit. The knowledge I accumulated, which I am so happy to be sharing with you, has already helped many people that share your desires and some of this knowledge has been well known and used successfully for centuries before it became known to me. You will now use this knowledge as well and what a great gift to your health and wellbeing your commitment to help yourself will be! **Investing in acquiring and then using the knowledge to help your body cells is the best investment you can ever make!** Let's start this journey together as I am here to help you understand what your blood cells would tell you right now if they could speak to you.

Chapter 1

The relationship between Acidity and active Cancer Cells

*I have found that **if you love life, life will love you back-***

Arthur Rubinstein

Let me first explain the nature of cancer cells and what causes them to become active or inactive in the tissues of the human body. It is a fact that everyone on planet Earth has cancer cells in their body. What we will recognize is that the cancer cells only become active and a threat to our tissues and organs when an acidic environment in our bodies develops. An acidic body environment allows the cancer cells to multiply and grow. Once we understand this, we can then focus our food and nutrition knowledge toward providing our bodies with the support it needs to remove and prevent active cancer cells within our bodies.

If we control the cancer cell environment in our body, we can control, beat and prevent cancer.

In detail, as this is so really important for you to understand and use effectively to empower and strengthen your body's defensive mechanisms, I am now going to spend some time explaining how you are going to deprive your cancer cells of the acidic environment within your body that they have thrived on so far.

First, as to the important question why some tissues in the body become prone to cancer, it is helpful to understand the nature, causes and effects of tissue **acidity** and **alkalinity** levels and how critical this is to the natural body defensive mechanisms our cells and tissues rely on.

Cancer prone tissues are those that have become more **acidic**, whereas **healthy tissues** remain within the normal **alkaline levels that the body needs**. Optimum alkalinity levels depend on **correct oxygen levels in the body, which help to neutralize acidity**, while, conversely, abnormal acidity levels prevent oxygen from reaching the tissues that need it. When tissues become devoid of free oxygen, acidity levels rise within the tissue which can then activate otherwise dormant cancer cells.

Alkalinity is just the reverse and allows oxygen into the tissues. The most important task you will be focusing on with the knowledge you find in this book is how you can create and maintain a **more alkaline environment** in your body. You will learn how you can continuously nurture this alkaline environment so that your body makes and keeps **cancer cells inactive**.

The way I explain this in more detail, is to talk in terms of the significance of the pH level of the body and of the pH level of the different foods that we put into our bodies. Relative to what our bodies required pH levels are, you will understand which foods have more **alkalinity** values and therefore more **cancer beating power** for our blood cells and tissues than those foods which are more acidic and which, if allowed to continue to be part of our normal diet, will allow cancer cells to continue to be active and potentially multiply.

The pH scale measures how acidic or alkaline a substance is and ranges from 0 to 14, with 7 being neutral. For this discussion, pH readings below 7 are **acidic** and above 7 are considered **alkaline**.

You are probably wondering what your body's healthy state pH level should be and what it is currently. The fact is that blood, lymph and cerebral spinal fluid in the human body are designed to be, and stay healthy in, an alkaline environment at a pH level of 7.4 or higher.

"At a pH level slightly above 7.4 cancer cells within our body become dormant and at the more alkaline level of pH 8.5, cancer cells will actually die while healthy cells will live" (Barefoot, pages 66-67).

This knowledge has given rise to the development of a variety of nutritional based regimens designed to increase the alkalinity of the body's tissues through:

1. The intake of specifically alkaline **vegetarian foods**
2. The drinking of alkalizing **fresh fruit and vegetable juices**
3. Foods particularly rich in **alkaline minerals** include **calcium, potassium, magnesium, caesium, rubidium, sodium, and selenium** as well as **antioxidant vitamins**.

I hope you are now at a point where you are really excited that you have, within your grasp, the knowledge and motivation to power your body back to health. You should now commence, as soon as possible, taking the steps to help your body to **become alkaline** and to **stay that way** so that your blood cells and tissues actually **have the power to neutralize the cancer cells in your body**. How to do that and to understand what kind of foods create the most acidity in the body you are going to learn the details of as you read my book. You now can appreciate that you should start eating more foods that have pH levels higher than neutral 7, while permanently eliminating foods from your diet that have pH levels of less than 7. Your best help for your body will result from a focused daily regimen of buying, cooking and eating the right foods to allow your body to disarm your cancer cells and put them into "hibernation" permanently.

Incredibly, much of the food we like and find in our local grocery store is actually dangerously acidic to our body tissues. Who would have expected for example, that **oranges that taste** so delicious and which are universally popular, have a pH level of **3.69 - 4.34**, which is <u>very acidic</u> and which unfortunately, in conjunction with other acidic foods, encourages cancer cells to become active and multiply. The same circumstances are true with tomatoes, particularly those that are eaten before they are properly ripened.

As you are now at the point where you will want to help your system as much as possible, **the tables you will read below will allow you to be clearly and quickly informed, and** to make the decision to say **NO** to the vegetables and fruits that do not help the body stay within its normal alkalinity range. Your blood cells are craving for you to give them a healthier environment and you can satisfy their needs once you have studied the information contained in this book.

We have to make and keep your system **optimally alkaline** by enabling you to replace the **acidic foods** in your diet with foods that are **alkaline as well as being delicious to your taste buds.** You can start helping your body today with delicious alternatives to select from which will allow you to continue to enjoy your food every day!

Some "borderline" neutral pH vegetables and fruits are acceptable to eat when they are fully ripe and grown organically and it is so indicated opposite each one in the table below. Later, I will also explain why it is so important for you to consume **organic** alkaline foods as much as possible and most probably you already know many of the reasons.

Earlier I mentioned the importance of foods rich in alkaline minerals. Here is a quote from Dr. Warburg and Dr. Brewer's research that shows the importance of alkaline minerals and how they work within cancer cells.

"*A mass spectrographic analysis of cancer cells showed that the cell membrane readily attached* **caesium, rubidium and potassium**, *and transmitted these elements with their associated molecules* **into the cancer cell***. In contrast cancer membranes did not transmit sodium, magnesium, and calcium into the cell: the amount of calcium within a cancer cell is only about 1% of that for normal cells.* **Potassium** *transports glucose into the cell.* **Calcium** *and* **magnesium** *transport* **oxygen** *into the cell. As a consequence of the above, oxygen cannot enter cancer cells so the glucose which is normally burned to carbon dioxide and water undergoes fermentation* **to form lactic acid** *within the cell.*"

Dr Warburg pointed out this anaerobic condition, **as early as 1924.**

"***Potassium*** *and especially* **rubidium** *and* **caesium** *are the most basic of the elements. When the cancer cells take them up they will thus* **raise the pH of the cells***. Since they are very strong bases as compared to the* **weak lactic acid** *it is possible that the pH will be raised to values in* **the 8.5 to 9 ranges***. In this range* **the life of the cancer cell is short***, being a matter of* **days** *at the most. The* **dead cancer cells** *are then absorbed by the body fluids and eventually eliminated from the system.*" – **Dr Brewer.**

15

There is research indicating that cancer grows slowly in a **highly acid environment** (because the **acids** cause it to **partially** destroy itself) and may actually grow more quickly as your body becomes more alkaline **prior to** reaching **the healthy pH slightly above 7.4 where the cancer becomes dormant.**

Therefore, you will want to raise your **pH above 7.4 as quickly as possible** by every means available. Once you have achieved a pH above 7.4, it is useful to monitor your saliva and urine pH regularly to ensure that your body remains **sufficiently alkaline**.

The Saliva PH test is a simple test you can do to measure your susceptibility to cancer, heart disease, osteoporosis, arthritis, and many other degenerative diseases. Buy your Saliva pH test kit from your local drug store or pharmacy.

How to Perform the Saliva pH Test

First, you must wait at least 2 hours after eating. Fill your mouth with saliva and then swallow it. Repeat this step to help ensure that your saliva is clean. Then after the third swallow, put some of your saliva onto the **pH paper**.

The pH paper should turn blue. This indicates that your saliva is slightly alkaline at a healthy pH of 7.4. If it is not blue, compare the colour with the chart that comes with the **pH paper**. If your saliva is acid (below pH of 7.0) wait two hours and repeat the test.

"When healthy, the pH of blood is 7.4, the pH of spinal fluid is 7.4, and the pH of saliva is 7.4. Thus the pH of saliva parallels the extra cellular fluid...pH test of saliva represents the most consistent and most definitive physical sign of the ionic calcium and other alkaline minerals deficiency syndrome...The pH of the non-deficient and healthy person is in the 7.5 (dark blue) to 7.1 (blue) slightly alkaline range. The range from 6.5 (blue-green), which is weakly acidic to 4.5 (light yellow) which is strongly acidic, represents alkalinity states from mildly deficient to strongly deficient, respectively."

To reiterate, as this is key to achieving a cancer resistant body environment and so very important, I recommend that you start:

I. **Alkalizing your body quickly by consistently eating the right foods and drinks**
II. **Eliminating all food that contains too much acidity from your diet.**

The chart below shows you the **most common acidic foods** that many of us consume every day without ever knowing the damage these foods inflict on our blood cells and tissues.

List of foods to avoid because they contain TOO much ACIDITY:

Tomatoes	**ACIDITY LEVEL:** **4.30 - 4.90** Consumable when grown organically and completely ripe
Sweet peppers	**ACIDITY LEVEL:** **4.65 - 5.45**
Red beetroots	**ACIDITY LEVEL:** **5.30 - 6.60**

Sorrel	**ACIDITY LEVEL:** **4.5**
Oranges	**ACIDITY LEVEL:** **3.69 - 4.34**
Mandarins, tangerines	**ACIDITY LEVEL:** **3.32 - 4.48**
Grapefruits	**ACIDITY LEVEL:** **3.00 - 3.75**

Strawberries	**ACIDITY LEVEL:**
	3.00 - 3.90 Consumable when grown organically and ripe
Raspberries	**ACIDITY LEVEL:**
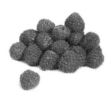	**3.22 - 3.95** Consumable when grown organically and ripe
Black-currant	**ACIDITY LEVEL:**
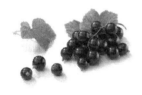	**4.8 – 7.0** Consumable when grown organically and ripe
Red-currant	**ACIDITY LEVEL:**
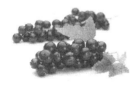	**4.8 – 7.0** Consumable when grown organically and ripe

Gooseberries	**ACIDITY LEVEL:** **2.80 - 3.10**
Pineapples	**ACIDITY LEVEL:** **3.20 - 4.00**
Kiwis	**ACIDITY LEVEL:** **3.1 – 3.96**
Dates	**ACIDITY LEVEL:** **4.14 - 4.88**

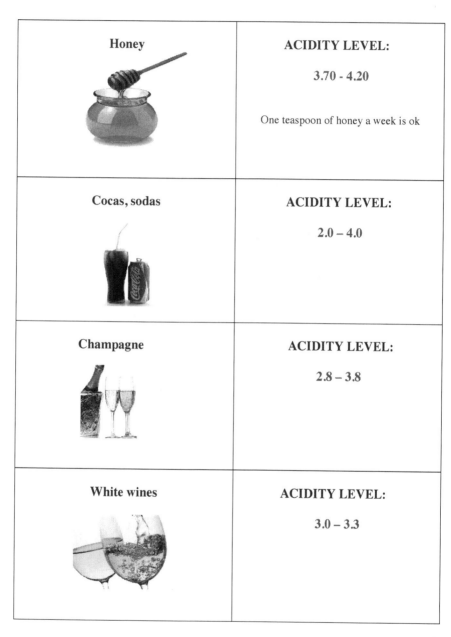

Honey	**ACIDITY LEVEL:** **3.70 - 4.20** One teaspoon of honey a week is ok
Cocas, sodas	**ACIDITY LEVEL:** **2.0 – 4.0**
Champagne	**ACIDITY LEVEL:** **2.8 – 3.8**
White wines	**ACIDITY LEVEL:** **3.0 – 3.3**

Pink wines 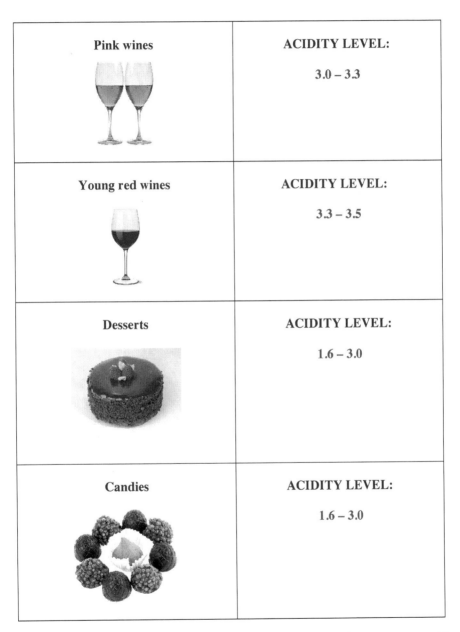	**ACIDITY LEVEL:** 3.0 – 3.3
Young red wines	**ACIDITY LEVEL:** 3.3 – 3.5
Desserts	**ACIDITY LEVEL:** 1.6 – 3.0
Candies	**ACIDITY LEVEL:** 1.6 – 3.0

Vinegar	ACIDITY LEVEL: 2.40 - 3.40
Pickles	ACIDITY LEVEL: 5.10 - 5.40

Chapter 2

How to Alkalize your Body

*"We delight in the **beauty** of the **butterfly**, but **rarely admit** the **changes** it has gone through **to achieve that beauty**."*

Maya Angelou

The **best** and the **quickest way** to **alkalize** your body will be for you to consistently eat, on a daily basis, fresh, preferably organic vegetables, fruits and other foods that contain plenty of **alkalizing minerals** and **antioxidant vitamins (these are cancer preventatives and have cancer cell destroying properties). As far as beverages are concerned,** drinking alkalizing fresh fruit & vegetable Juices that you can get at your local health store will further reduce the time it takes you to reach the level of alkalinity your body needs to defeat cancer.

Before we look at the alkalizing food charts and tables that will become your "go to" guide for what to select for your every day alkalizing nutrients and minerals, I want to strongly recommend to you a **SUPER ALKALINE juice or pill supplement known as "Wheatgrass"** which I can't emphasize enough to you as one that you should search out immediately and take on a daily basis, preferably via **shots of fresh wheatgrass juice** on its own or mixed into your fruit juice according to your taste preferences.

WHEATGRASS IS ONE OF THE BEST ALKALINITY SOURCES

*"When we **love**, we always strive to become **better** than we are. When we strive **to become better** than we are, everything around us **becomes better too**."*

Paulo Coelho, the Alchemist

WHEATGRASS JUICE...

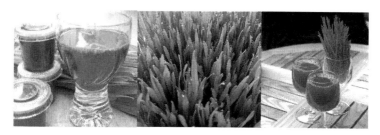

Wheatgrass is so important for you at this time as it has the amazing ability to cleanse the blood, organs and gastrointestinal tract of **debris** and **toxins**; it **increases the red blood-cell count** and lowers blood pressure! Wheatgrass stimulates your **metabolism** and the body's **enzyme systems** by enriching the blood. It also aids in reducing blood pressure by dilating the blood pathways throughout the body.

Wheatgrass fights tumors and neutralizes toxins.

Recent studies show that wheatgrass juice has a powerful ability to **fight tumors** without the usual toxicity of drugs that also inhibit cell-destroying agents. The many active compounds found in wheatgrass juice cleanse the blood and neutralize and digest toxins in our cells.

As you know chemotherapy and radiation treatments as well as killing cancer cells, produce a lot of toxins and destroy a lot healthy cells and this is where **wheatgrass** comes as a huge **rejuvenating** and detoxifying tool.

The enzymes and amino acids found in wheatgrass can protect us from carcinogens like no other food or medicine. **It strengthens our cells**, **detoxifies** the **liver** and bloodstream, and chemically neutralizes environmental pollutants.

Restores alkalinity to the blood. The juice's abundance of **alkaline minerals** helps **reduce over-acidity** in the blood. It can be used to relieve many internal pains, and has been used successfully to treat peptic ulcers, ulcerative colitis, constipation, diarrhea, and other complaints of the gastrointestinal tract.

Wheatgrass is a **concentrated** source of many nutrients, especially **Beta-carotene (Vitamin A), Calcium, Iron, Vitamin K, Vitamin C, Vitamin B12, Folic acid, Vitamin B6** and other trace nutrients.

Wheatgrass has a remarkable similarity to our own blood. Wheatgrass Juice is one of the best sources of **living chlorophyll available**. It contains **70% chlorophyll,** chlorophyll being the basis of all plant life.

Science has proven that chlorophyll **arrests growth** and **development** of unfriendly bacteria and helps to destroy **free radicals. Chlorophyll (wheatgrass juice)** has a nearly identical chemical structure to **hemoglobin (red blood cells),** which is the body's **critical oxygen** and **iron-carrying** blood protein. Dr. Birscher, a research scientist, called chlorophyll **"Concentrated Sun Power."** He says chlorophyll **increases** function of the **heart,** affects the **vascular system**, the **uterus**, the **intestine** and the **lungs**. According to Dr. Birscher, nature uses chlorophyll as a **body cleanser**, **rebuilder** and **neutralizer of toxins**.

Dr. Yoshihide Hagiwara, president of the Hagiwara Institute of Health in Japan, is a leading advocate for the use of wheatgrass as **food** and **medicine**. He reasons that since chlorophyll is soluble in fat particles, and fat particles are absorbed directly into the blood via the lymphatic system, that chlorophyll can also be absorbed in this way. In other words, when the "blood" of plants is absorbed in humans it is transformed into human blood, which transports nutrients to **every cell of the body**.

Wheatgrass offers the benefits of a liquid oxygen transfusion since the juice contains liquid oxygen. **Oxygen** is vital to many body processes: it stimulates **digestion** (the oxidation of food), promotes **clearer thinking** (the brain utilizes 25% of the body's oxygen supply), and protects the blood against anaerobic bacteria. **Cancer cells cannot exist in the presence of oxygen**.

Interestingly, Wheatgrass has been found to turn grey hair to its natural color again and greatly increases energy levels, when consumed daily.

Please don't cook it. We can only get the benefits of the many enzymes found in wheatgrass by eating it uncooked. Cooking destroys **100 percent** of the **enzymes** that are so vital for us in food.

Wheatgrass can also:

- **Neutralize toxic substances** like cadmium, nicotine, strontium, mercury, and polyvinyl chloride.

- **Lessen the effects of radiation**. One enzyme found in wheatgrass, SOD, lessens the effects of radiation and acts as an anti-inflammatory compound that may **prevent cellular damage** following **heart attacks** or exposure to irritants.

- **Double your red blood cell count** just by soaking in it. You can apply fresh wheatgrass juice to the face for 15-20 min and see the results after using it just a few times. Renowned nutritionist Dr. Bernard Jensen found that **no other blood builders** are superior to **green juices** and **wheatgrass**. In his book Health Magic Through Chlorophyll from Living Plant Life he mentions several cases where he was able to **double the red blood cell count** in a matter **of days** merely by having patients soak in a chlorophyll-water bath. **Blood building results** occur even more rapidly when patients drink green juices and wheatgrass regularly.

Detoxification is the process of reducing the "**body burden**" by **eliminating toxins** that have been building for years or even decades. Because of the presence of **chlorophyll,** wheatgrass juice will cause detoxification to take place. If your body has stored toxins, it will Detox.

If you Detox too quickly, it is possible to have side effects that cause you to **temporarily** feel worse. When toxins re-enter the bloodstream, they can trigger an immune response that is termed a "healing crisis". This is a natural process, but can be uncomfortable and may include symptoms such as a headache (particularly for high sugar consumers, which I am sure you are avoiding now), flu-like feelings, diarrhea or fatigue. A healing crisis is not desirable and in most cases not necessary. If you have time, start with a small amount of juice and work your way up to avoid this experience. It is necessary to drink plenty of water when detoxing, approximately 2 - 2.5 L a day. It's also very important not to drink any cold water or other drinks with meals; you should stop drinking water 15 min before a meal and start drinking 40-45 min after a meal (due to the quality of digestion). If Detox is noticeable, recognize it as a positive sign, consider reducing your juice consumption temporarily and be confident that it will pass. In a short period of time (1 day for some, less than 1 week for most, 1 month in rare circumstances) your body will be cleansed and you will experience the **mental clarity** and physical **rejuvenation** that comes with **wheatgrass juice.**

As you can see, fresh wheatgrass juice (or any form available) will help you enormously to cope with chemotherapy side effects by **neutralizing chemicals** and **toxins**, increasing your **red blood cell** count, fighting with **tumors**, providing more **oxygen** to the cells and to the brain. All this is very critical and necessary help that you can provide for your body right now.

Suggested Dosage:

For normal health maintenance -1 to 4 oz. daily;
For therapeutic dosage - 4 to 8 oz. daily;
In **crisis** - 10 oz. daily.

Wheatgrass is a powerful "detoxifier" of both the liver and large intestine. Consequently, people should gradually increase from **one ounce** a day to **eight ounces** spread throughout the day.

Recommended duration: 60 days.

Traditionally, it is taken on an empty stomach, at least 15 minutes before a meal.

We also have available from Mother Nature another **Super Antioxidant**: **"Chia Seeds"** that I would like you to add as a second daily dietary supplement with your wheatgrass juice shots:

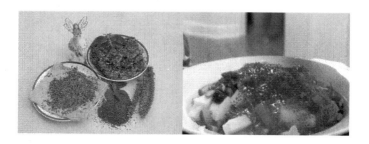

Chia is an astonishingly powerful **natural seed**. In 2008, a study by the Department of Foods and Nutrition, Purdue University, Indiana, USA reported that Chia contained, among other things, **significant amounts of antioxidants**.

Chia's army of antioxidants include flavonol aglycones: quercetin, kaempferol, and myricetin; and flavonol glycosides: **chlorogenic acid** and **caffeic acid**. These antioxidants have significant value to **human health.**

There are also reports saying that the **black Chia seeds** may contain 12%-15% more antioxidants that the **white seeds**. A study by the US-based Nutritional Science Research Institute performed a study on Chia seeds.

"... Chia seeds as one of the most powerful, whole food antioxidant we know."

32

Antioxidants contained in Chia seeds

Quercetin, one of Chia's **powerful antioxidants**, has been at the top of recent health news. Early this year, a study by researchers at the University of South Carolina's Arnold School of Public Health shows that *quercetin* significantly boosted energy, endurance and fitness in healthy men and women who were not involved in some type of daily physical training. This means that this antioxidant's fatigue-fighting properties could help average adults who battle fatigue and stress daily.

Quercetin, kaempferol, and *myricetin* are **antioxidants** that could protect against a host of chronic diseases like **ischemic heart disease**, cerebrovascular disease, **lung cancer**, **prostate cancer**, asthma, and **diabetes**.

Chlorogenic Acid, another of Chia's **antioxidants**, has been found by a study to possess **anti-cancer properties** and could be used to prevent growth of certain **brain tumors**. It could also slow the release of glucose into bloodstream after a meal, and is a compound of interest for reducing the risk of developing Type 2 Diabetes. *Chlorogenic acids* do other things too: help the flow of bile, thus reducing bile stagnation and promoting **liver** and **gallbladder health**. It could also help to reduce cardiovascular risks. The body easily absorbs its nutritional benefits if it was sourced from natural, whole foods.

Caffeic acid, another antioxidant in Chia, may be used as a component to contribute to the prevention of the following: colitis, a condition that could lead to colon cancer, cardiovascular disease, **certain cancers,** mitosis (cell division) and inflammation. It may also be used in the healthy maintenance of the **immune system.**

Antioxidants in Chia seeds and oil help prevent cancer:

The most important antioxidants contained in Chia seeds are **chlorgenic acid** and **caffeic acid.** These are antioxidants that play a major role in **cancer prevention** and fighting **free radicals**.

Omega-3s

Chia seeds are the highest plant source of omega-3s. Omega-3s are healthy fatty acids that are needed for normal body and **brain functioning**, hormonal balance and the **absorption** of essential vitamins. Chia seeds consist of approximately 60 to 65 percent omega-3s, making them a potent **anti-inflammatory food**. Furthermore, since Chia seeds are a whole food and rich in antioxidants, they maintain freshness longer than most other sources of omega-3s such as fish oils and hemp seeds.

Recommended Doses:

Chia seeds are unique in that there is no recommended dosage or evidence of risks from possibly eating too much.

The amount used varies among individuals, how they feel and their needs. Adults consuming Chia for general nutrition and health purposes, such as increased energy, might typically consume 2 tbsp. per day.

100 grams (3.5oz.) of Omega^3 Chia is:

• a source of **Magnesium** equivalent to 53 ounces of Broccoli

• a source of **Iron** equivalent to 10 ounces of Spinach

• a source of **Folate** equivalent to 2 ounces of Asparagus

• a source of **Fiber** equivalent to 4 ounces of Bran

• a source of **Calcium** equivalent to 23 ounces of sesame seed

• a source of **Potassium** equivalent to 6 ounces of Bananas

• a source of **Antioxidants** equivalent to 10 ounces of Blueberries

• a source of **Omega3** Fatty Acids equivalent to 28 ounces of Atlantic Salmon

The above information shows you how rich Chia Seeds are in **alkalizing minerals** and full of **antioxidants** that can play a crucial role for you at this particular moment while you are on chemotherapy, helping to quickly provide an alkalizing effect for your system. Chia seeds will also be important generally in the future to help you to stay healthy.

Based on the knowledge you've already learned above let's build on your understanding of the **solutions and actions you can take now**.

The first and most important step is to get your system **alkalized as quickly as possible** and you can start doing it today! Apart from adding **wheatgrass juice** and **Chia seeds** to your daily diet, you should start eating organic vegetables, fruits, beans, peas, grains, seeds and nuts, which are full of **alkalizing minerals** and **antioxidant vitamins** as well as **cancer preventative enzymes**.

Please spend as much time as you need to carefully study the various tables below as these will be your "go to" reference tables on what to buy and eat to achieve and maintain optimum alkalinity for your body tissues.

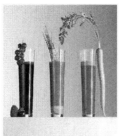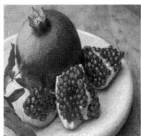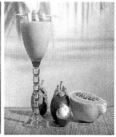

In summary, on a daily basis, you should be consuming alkaline vegetables that are shown in the chart below. The chart shows you how much **cancer preventative minerals** and **antioxidant vitamins** each vegetable contains. All vegetables shown below should be consumed when **ripe** and, ideally, having been **grown organically**.

*"The world as we have created it is **a process** of our thinking. It cannot be changed without changing our thinking."*

Albert Einstein

Best Alkalizing Vegetables with Mineral and Vitamin content details

Vegetable	Amount	Minerals Contained	Vitamins Contained
Alfalfa, sprouted	One cup of raw, sprouted alfalfa seeds contains 1.32 grams of protein, 8 calories and 0.6 grams of dietary fiber.	Potassium - 26 mg Phosphorus - 23 mg Magnesium - 9 mg Calcium - 11 mg Iron - 0.32 mg Sodium - 2 mg Zinc - 0.3 mg Copper - 0.052 mg Manganese - 0.062 mg Selenium - 0.2 mcg Also contains small amounts of other minerals.	Vitamin C - 2.7 mg Vitamin B1 (thiamine) - 0.025 mg Vitamin B2 (riboflavin) - 0.042 mg Niacin - 0.159 mg Pantothenic Acid - 0.186 mg Vitamin B6 - 0.011 mg Folate - 12 mcg Vitamin A - 51 IU Vitamin K - 10.1

			mcg Vitamin E - 0.01 mg Contains some other vitamins in small amounts.
Amaranth leaves 	One cup of amaranth leaves, cooked, boiled, drained with no added salt has 2.79 grams protein and 28 calories.	Potassium - 846 mg Phosphorus - 95 mg Magnesium - 73 mg Calcium - 276 mg Iron - 2.98 mg Zinc - 1.16 mg Manganese - 1.137 mg Sodium - 28 mg Copper - 0.209 mg Selenium - 1.2 mcg Also contains small amounts of other minerals.	Vitamin C - 54.3 mg Vitamin B1 (thiamine) - 0.026 mg Vitamin B2 (riboflavin) - 0.177 mg Niacin - 0.738 mg Pantothenic Acid - 0.082 mg Vitamin B6 - 0.234 mg Folate - 75 mcg Vitamin A - 3656 IU Contains some other vitamins in small amounts.
Artichoke 	One medium artichoke cooked with no added salt has 3.47 grams protein, 64 calories and 10.3 grams of fiber.	Potassium - 343 mg Phosphorus - 88 mg Magnesium - 50 mg Calcium - 25 mg Iron - 0.73 mg Zinc - 0.48 mg Copper - 0.152 mg Manganese - 0.27 mg Selenium - 0.2 mcg Sodium - 72 mg Also contains small amounts of other minerals.	Vitamin C - 8.9 mg Niacin - 1.332 mg Vitamin B1 (thiamine) - 0.06 mg Vitamin B2 (riboflavin) - 0.107 mg Vitamin B6 - 0.097 mg Pantothenic Acid - 0.288 mg Folate - 107 mcg Vitamin A - 16 IU Vitamin K - 17.8 mcg Vitamin E - 0.23 mg Contains some other vitamins in small amounts.
Asparagus	Half cup (about 6 spears) cooked with no added salt contains 2.16 grams of protein,	Potassium - 202 mg Phosphorus - 49 mg Calcium - 21 mg Iron - 0.82 mg Sodium - 13 mg	Vitamin A - 905 IU Vitamin C - 6.9 mg Niacin - 0.976 mg Vitamin B1 (thiamine) -

		Magnesium - 13 mg	0.146 mg
	20 calories and 1.8 grams of fiber.	Zinc - 0.54 mg Copper - 0.149 mg Manganese - 0.139 mg Selenium - 5.5 mcg Also contains small amounts of other minerals.	Vitamin B2 (riboflavin) - 0.125 mg Pantothenic Acid - 0.203 mg Vitamin B6 - 0.071 mg Folate - 134 mcg Vitamin K - 45.5 mcg Vitamin E - 1.35 mg Contains some other vitamins in small amounts.
Bamboo shoots 	One cup of bamboo shoots, cooked, boiled, drained with no added salt has 1.84 grams protein, 14 calories and 1.2 grams dietary fiber.	Potassium - 640 mg Phosphorus - 24 mg Magnesium - 4 mg Calcium - 14 mg Iron - 0.29 mg Sodium - 5 mg Zinc - 0.56 mg Copper - 0.098 mg Manganese - 0.136 mg Selenium - 0.5 mcg Also contains small amounts of other minerals.	Niacin - 0.36 mg Vitamin B1 (thiamine) - 0.024 mg Vitamin B2 (riboflavin) - 0.06 mg Pantothenic Acid - 0.079 mg Vitamin B6 - 0.118 mg Folate - 2 mcg Contains some other vitamins in small amounts.
Bok Choy 	One cup of Bok Choy (Pak Choi), cooked, boiled, drained with no added salt has 2.65 grams protein, 20 calories and 1.7 grams dietary fiber.	Potassium - 631 mg Phosphorus - 49 mg Magnesium - 19 mg Calcium - 158 mg Iron - 1.77 mg Zinc - 0.29 mg Copper - 0.032 mg Manganese - 0.245 mg Selenium - 0.7 mcg Sodium - 58 mg Also contains small amounts of other minerals.	Vitamin C - 44.2 mg Niacin - 0.728 mg Vitamin B1 (thiamine) - 0.054 mg Vitamin B2 (riboflavin) - 0.107 mg Pantothenic Acid - 0.134 mg Vitamin B6 - 0.282 mg Folate - 70 mcg Vitamin A - 7223 IU Vitamin E - 0.15 mg Vitamin K - 57.8 mcg Contains some other

			vitamins in small amounts.
Broccoli	Half cup of broccoli, cooked with no added salt contains 1.86 grams protein, 27 calories and 2.6 grams dietary fiber.	Potassium - 229 mg Phosphorus - 52 mg Calcium - 31 mg Sodium - 32 mg Magnesium - 16 mg Iron - 0.52 mg Zinc - 0.35 mg Copper - 0.048 mg Manganese - 0.151 mg Selenium - 1.2 mcg Also contains small amounts of other minerals.	Vitamin A - 1207 IU Vitamin C - 50.6 mg Niacin - 0.431 mg Vitamin B1 (thiamine) - 0.049 mg Vitamin B2 (riboflavin) - 0.096 mg Vitamin B6 - 0.156 mg Pantothenic Acid - 0.48 mg Folate - 84 mcg Vitamin K - 110 mcg Vitamin E - 1.13 mg Contains some other vitamins in small amounts.
Brussels Sprouts	One cup of Brussels Sprouts, cooked, boiled, drained with no added salt has 3.98 grams protein, 56 calories and 4.1 grams dietary fiber.	Potassium - 495 mg Phosphorus - 87 mg Magnesium - 31 mg Calcium - 56 mg Iron - 1.87 mg Zinc - 0.51 mg Copper - 0.129 mg Manganese - 0.354 mg Selenium - 2.3 mcg Sodium - 33 mg Also contains small amounts of other minerals.	Vitamin C - 96.7 mg Niacin - 0.947 mg Vitamin B1 (thiamine) - 0.167 mg Vitamin B2 (riboflavin) - 0.125 mg Pantothenic Acid - 0.393 mg Vitamin B6 - 0.278 mg Folate - 94 mcg Vitamin A - 1209 IU Vitamin E - 0.67 mg Vitamin K - 218.9 mcg Contains some other vitamins in small amounts.
Butternut squash	One cup of Butternut squash, cooked, baked,	Potassium - 582 mg Phosphorus - 55 mg Magnesium - 59 mg	Vitamin C - 31 mg Niacin - 1.986 mg Vitamin

	drained with no added salt has 1.84 grams protein and 82 calories.	Calcium - 84 mg Iron - 1.23 mg Zinc - 0.27 mg Copper - 0.133 mg Manganese - 0.353 mg Selenium - 1 mcg Sodium - 8 mg Also contains small amounts of other minerals.	B1 (thiamine) - 0.148 mg Vitamin B2 (riboflavin) - 0.035 mg Pantothenic Acid - 0.736 mg Vitamin B6 - 0.254 mg Folate - 39 mcg Vitamin A - 22868 IU Vitamin K - 2 mcg Vitamin E - 2.64 mg Contains some other vitamins in small amounts.
Cabbage 	One half cup of cabbage, cooked, boiled, drained with no added salt has 0.95 grams protein, 17 calories and 1.4 grams of dietary fiber.	Potassium - 147 mg Phosphorus - 25 mg Magnesium - 11 mg Calcium - 36 mg Iron - 0.13 mg Sodium - 6 mg Zinc - 0.15 mg Copper - 0.013 mg Manganese - 0.154 mg Selenium - 0.5 mcg Also contains small amounts of other minerals.	Vitamin C - 28.1 mg Niacin - 0.186 mg Vitamin B1 (thiamine) - 0.046 mg Vitamin B2 (riboflavin) - 0.029 mg Vitamin B6 - 0.084 mg Folate - 22 mcg Pantothenic Acid - 0.13 mg Vitamin A - 60 IU Vitamin K - 81.5 mcg Vitamin E - 0.11 mg Contains some other vitamins in small amounts.
Carrots 	Half cup cooked with no added salt contains 0.59 grams protein, 27 calories and 2.3 grams fiber.	Potassium - 183 mg Calcium - 23 mg Phosphorus - 23 mg Magnesium - 8 mg Iron - 0.27 mg Sodium - 5 mg Zinc - 0.3 mg Copper - 0.052 mg Manganese - 0.062 mg Selenium - 0.2 mcg Also contains small amounts of other	Vitamin A - 13286 IU Vitamin C - 2.8 mg Vitamin B1 (thiamine) - 0.051 mg Vitamin B2 (riboflavin) - 0.034 mg Niacin - 0.503 mg Folate - 11 mcg Pantothenic Acid -

			minerals.	0.181 mg Vitamin B6 - 0.119 mg Vitamin K - 10.7 mcg Vitamin E - 0.8 mg Contains some other vitamins in small amounts.
Cauliflower	Half cup cooked with no added salt contains 1.14 grams protein, 14 calories and 1.4 grams fiber.	Potassium - 88 mg Phosphorus - 20 mg Calcium - 10 mg Iron - 0.2 mg Magnesium - 6 mg Sodium - 9 mg Zinc - 0.11 mg Copper - 0.011 mg Manganese - 0.082 mg Selenium - 0.4 mcg Also contains small amounts of other minerals.	Vitamin C - 27.5 mg Niacin - 0.254 mg Vitamin B1 (thiamine) - 0.026 mg Vitamin B2 (riboflavin) - 0.032 mg Folate - 27 mcg Vitamin B6 - 0.107 mg Pantothenic Acid - 0.315 mg Vitamin A - 7 IU Vitamin K - 8.6 mcg Vitamin E - 0.04 mg Contains some other vitamins in small amounts.
Celeriac	One cup of Celeriac, cooked, boiled, drained with no added salt has 1.49 grams protein, 42 calories and 1.9 grams of dietary fiber.	Potassium - 268 mg Phosphorus - 102 mg Magnesium - 19 mg Calcium - 40 mg Iron - 0.67 mg Sodium - 95 mg Zinc - 0.31 mg Copper - 0.067 mg Manganese - 0.149 mg Selenium - 0.6 mcg Also contains small amounts of other minerals.	Vitamin C - 5.6 mg Niacin - 0.662 mg Vitamin B1 (thiamine) - 0.042 mg Vitamin B2 (riboflavin) - 0.057 mg Vitamin B6 - 0.157 mg Folate - 5 mcg Pantothenic Acid - 0.315 mg Contains some other vitamins in small amounts.
Celery	One cup of celery, cooked, boiled, drained with no added salt	Potassium - 426 mg Phosphorus - 38 mg Magnesium - 18 mg Calcium - 63 mg	Vitamin C - 9.2 mg Niacin - 0.479 mg Vitamin B1 (thiamine) -

	has 1.25 grams protein, 27 calories and 2.4 grams of dietary fiber.	Iron - 0.63 mg Sodium - 136 mg Zinc - 0.21 mg Copper - 0.054 mg Manganese - 0.159 mg Selenium - 1.5 mcg Also contains small amounts of other minerals.	0.064 mg Vitamin B2 (riboflavin) - 0.07 mg Vitamin B6 - 0.129 mg Folate - 33 mcg Pantothenic Acid - 0.292 mg Vitamin A - 782 IU Vitamin K - 56.7 mcg Vitamin E - 0.53 IU Contains some other vitamins in small amounts.
Chinese broccoli 	One cup of Chinese broccoli, cooked, boiled, drained with no added salt has 1 gram protein, 19 calories and 2.2 grams of dietary fiber.	Potassium - 230 mg Phosphorus - 36 mg Magnesium - 16 mg Calcium - 88 mg Iron - 0.49 mg Sodium - 6 mg Zinc - 0.34 mg Copper - 0.054 mg Manganese - 0.232 mg Selenium - 1.1 mcg Also contains small amounts of other minerals.	Vitamin C - 24.8 mg Niacin - 0.385 mg Vitamin B1 (thiamine) - 0.084 mg Vitamin B2 (riboflavin) - 0.128 mg Vitamin B6 - 0.062 mg Folate - 87 mcg Pantothenic Acid - 0.14 mg Vitamin A - 1441 IU Vitamin K - 74.6 mcg Vitamin E - 0.42 mg Contains some other vitamins in small amounts.
Chinese cabbage 	One cup of Chinese cabbage (pe-tsai), cooked, boiled, drained with no added salt has 1.78 grams protein, 17 calories and 2 grams of dietary fiber.	Potassium - 268 mg Phosphorus - 46 mg Magnesium - 12 mg Calcium - 38 mg Iron - 0.36 mg Sodium - 11 mg Zinc - 0.21 mg Copper - 0.035 mg Manganese - 0.182 mg Selenium - 0.5 mcg Also contains small amounts of other	Vitamin C - 18.8 mg Niacin - 0.595 mg Vitamin B1 (thiamine) - 0.052 mg Vitamin B2 (riboflavin) - 0.052 mg Vitamin B6 - 0.0211 mg Folate - 63 mcg Pantothenic Acid -

		minerals.	0.095 mg Vitamin A - 1151 IU Contains some other vitamins in small amounts.
Corn	One large ear of yellow corn, cooked with no salt contains 4.02 grams protein, 113 calories and 2.8 grams fiber.	Potassium - 257 mg Phosphorus - 91 mg Magnesium - 31 mg Calcium - 4 mg Selenium - 0.2 mg Iron - 0.53 mg Zinc - 0.73 mg Copper - 0.058 mg Manganese - 0.197 mg Also contains small amounts of other minerals.	Vitamin C - 6.5 mg Niacin - 1.986 mg Vitamin B1 (thiamine) - 0.11 mg Vitamin B2 (riboflavin) - 0.067 mg Vitamin B6 - 0.164 mg Folate - 27 mcg Pantothenic Acid - 0.935 mg Vitamin A - 310 IU Vitamin K - 0.5 mcg Vitamin E - 0.11 mg Contains some other vitamins in small amounts.
Cucumber	Half a cup of sliced cucumber with skins contains .34 grams protein, 8 calories and .3 grams fiber.	Potassium - 76 mg Phosphorus - 12 mg Magnesium - 7 mg Sodium - 1 mg Calcium - 8 mg Iron - 0.15 mg Zinc - 0.1 mg Copper - 0.021 mg Manganese - 0.041 mg Selenium - 0.2 mcg Also contains small amounts of other minerals.	Vitamin C - 1.5 mg Niacin - 0.051 mg Vitamin B1 (thiamine) - 0.014 mg Vitamin B2 (riboflavin) - 0.017 mg Vitamin B6 - 0.021 mg Folate - 4 mcg Pantothenic Acid - 0.135 mg Vitamin A - 55 IU Vitamin K - 8.5 mcg Vitamin E - 0.02 mg Contains some other vitamins in small amounts.
Daikon Radish	One cup of Daikon Radish(oriental),	Potassium - 419 mg Phosphorus - 35 mg Magnesium - 13 mg	Vitamin C - 22.2 mg Niacin - 0.221 mg

	cooked, boiled, drained with no added salt has 0.98 grams protein, 25 calories and 2.4 grams of dietary fiber.	Calcium - 25 mg Iron - 0.22 mg < Sodium - 19 mg Zinc - 0.19 mg Copper - 0.148 mg Manganese - 0.049 mg Selenium - 1 mcg Also contains small amounts of other minerals.	Vitamin B2 (riboflavin) - 0.034 mg Vitamin B6 - 0.056 mg Folate - 25 mcg Pantothenic Acid - 0.168 mg Vitamin K - 0.4 mcg Contains some other vitamins in small amounts.
Eggplant	One cup of eggplant, cooked, boiled, drained with no added salt has 0.82 grams protein, 35 calories and 2.5 grams of dietary fiber.	Potassium - 122 mg Phosphorus - 15 mg Magnesium - 11 mg Calcium - 6 mg Iron - 0.25 mg Sodium - 1 mg Zinc - 0.12 mg Copper - 0.058 mg Manganese - 0.112 mg Selenium - 0.1 mcg Also contains small amounts of other minerals.	Vitamin C - 1.3 mg Niacin - 0.594 mg Vitamin B1 (thiamine) - 0.075 mg Vitamin B2 (riboflavin) - 0.02 mg Vitamin B6 - 0.085 mg Folate - 14 mcg Pantothenic Acid - 0.074 mg Vitamin A - 37 IU Vitamin K - 2.9 mcg Vitamin E - 0.41 mg Contains some other vitamins in small amounts.
Fennel	One cup of raw fennel bulb has 1.08 grams protein, 27 calories and 2.7 grams of dietary fiber.	Potassium - 360 mg Phosphorus - 44 mg Magnesium - 15 mg Calcium - 43 mg Iron - 0.64 mg Sodium - 45 mg Zinc - 0.17 mg Copper - 0.057 mg Manganese - 0.166 mg Selenium - 0.6 mcg Also contains small amounts of other minerals.	Vitamin C - 10.4 mg Niacin - 0.557 mg Vitamin B1 (thiamine) - 0.009 mg Vitamin B2 (riboflavin) - 0.028 mg Vitamin B6 - 0.041 mg Folate - 23 mcg Pantothenic Acid - 0.202 mg Vitamin A - 117 IU Contains some other vitamins in small

			amounts.
French beans 	One cup of French beans, mature seeds, cooked, boiled with no added salt has 12.48 grams protein, 228 calories and 16.6 grams of dietary fiber.	Potassium - 655 mg Phosphorus - 181 mg Magnesium - 99 mg Calcium - 112 mg Iron - 1.91 mg Sodium - 11 mg Zinc - 1.13 mg Copper - 0.204 mg Manganese - 0.676 mg Selenium - 2.1 mcg Also contains small amounts of other minerals.	Vitamin C - 2.1 mg Niacin - 0.966 mg Vitamin B1 (thiamine) - 0.23 mg Vitamin B2 (riboflavin) - 0.11 mg Vitamin B6 - 0.186 mg Folate - 133 mcg Pantothenic Acid - 0.393 mg Vitamin A - 5 IU Contains some other vitamins in small amounts.
Jicama 	One hundred grams of jicama, cooked or boiled with no added salt has 0.72 grams protein and 38 calories.	Potassium - 135 mg Phosphorus - 16 mg Magnesium - 11 mg Calcium - 11 mg Iron - 0.57 mg Sodium - 4 mg Zinc - 0.15 mg Copper - 0.046 mg Manganese - 0.057 mg Selenium - 0.7 mcg Also contains small amounts of other minerals.	Vitamin C - 14.1 mg Niacin - 0.19 mg Vitamin B1 (thiamine) - 0.017 mg Vitamin B2 (riboflavin) - 0.028 mg Vitamin B6 - 0.04 mg Folate - 8 mcg Pantothenic Acid - 0.121 mg Vitamin A - 19 IU Contains some other vitamins in small amounts.
Kale 	One cup of cooked kale with no added salt contains 2.47 grams protein, 36 calories and 2.6 grams fiber.	Potassium - 296 mg Phosphorus - 36 mg Magnesium - 23 mg Calcium - 94 mg Iron - 1.17 mg Sodium - 30 mg Zinc - 0.31 mg Copper - 0.203 mg Manganese - 0.541 mg Selenium - 1.2 mcg Also contains small amounts of other minerals.	Vitamin A - 17,707 IU Vitamin C - 53.3 mg Niacin - 0.65 mg Vitamin B1 (thiamine) - 0.069 mg Vitamin B2 (riboflavin) - 0.091 mg Vitamin B6 - 0.179 mg

			Folate - 17 mcg Pantothenic Acid - 0.064 mg Vitamin K - 1062 mcg Vitamin E - 1.1 mg Contains some other vitamins in small amounts.
Leek 	One leek, cooked, boiled with no added salt has 1 gram protein, 38 calories and 1.2 grams of dietary fiber.	Potassium - 108 mg Phosphorus - 21 mg Magnesium - 17 mg Calcium - 37 mg Iron - 1.36 mg Sodium - 12 mg Zinc - 0.07 mg Copper - 0.077 mg Manganese - 0.306 mg Selenium - 0.6 mcg Also contains small amounts of other minerals.	Vitamin C - 5.2 mg Niacin - 0.248 mg Vitamin B1 (thiamine) - 0.032 mg Vitamin B2 (riboflavin) - 0.025 mg Vitamin B6 - 0.14 mg Folate - 30 mcg Pantothenic Acid - 0.089 mg Vitamin A - 1007 IU Vitamin K - 31.5 mcg Vitamin E - 0.62 mg Contains some other vitamins in small amounts.
Lima Beans 	One cup of cooked large lima beans with no added salt contains 14.66 grams protein, 216 calories and 13.2 grams fiber.	Potassium - 955 mg Phosphorus - 209 mg Magnesium - 81 mg Calcium - 32 mg Selenium - 8.5 mg Iron - 4.49 mg Sodium - 4 mg Zinc - 1.79 mg Manganese - 0.97 mg Copper - 0.442 mg Also contains small amounts of other minerals.	Pantothenic Acid - 0.793 mg Niacin - 0.791 mg Vitamin B1 (thiamine) - 0.303 mg Vitamin B2 (riboflavin) - 0.103 mg Vitamin B6 - 0.303 mg Folate - 156 mcg Vitamin K - 3.8 mcg Vitamin E - 0.34 mg Contains some other vitamins in small amounts.

Mushroom	Half a cup of raw mushrooms contains 1.08 grams of protein, 8 calories and 0.3 grams of fiber.	Potassium - 111 mg Phosphorus - 30 mg Magnesium - 3 mg Calcium - 1 mg Iron - 0.17 mg Sodium - 2 mg Zinc - 0.18 mg Copper - 0.111 mg Manganese - 0.016 mg Selenium - 3.3 mcg Also contains small amounts of other minerals.	Vitamin D - 2 IU Niacin - 1.262 mg Vitamin B1 (thiamine) - 0.028 mg Vitamin B2 (riboflavin) - 0.141 mg Vitamin B6 - 0.036 mg Vitamin C - 0.7 mg Pantothenic Acid - 0.524 mg Folate - 6 mcg Contains some other vitamins in small amounts.
Okra	One cup of okra, cooked, boiled, drained, with no added salt has 3 grams protein, 35 calories and 4 grams of dietary fiber.	Potassium - 216 mg Phosphorus - 51 mg Magnesium - 58 mg Calcium - 123 mg Iron - 0.45 mg Sodium - 10 mg Zinc - 0.69 mg Copper - 0.136 mg Manganese - 0.47 mg Selenium - 0.6 mcg Also contains small amounts of other minerals.	Vitamin C - 26.1 mg Niacin - 1.394 mg Vitamin B1 (thiamine) - 0.211 mg Vitamin B2 (riboflavin) - 0.088 mg Vitamin B6 - 0.299 mg Folate - 74 mcg Pantothenic Acid - 0.341 mg Vitamin A - 453 IU Vitamin K - 64 mcg Vitamin E - 0.43 mg Contains some other vitamins in small amounts.
Onions	One small onion cooked without salt contains 0.82 grams protein, 26 calories and 0.8 grams of fiber.	Potassium - 100 mg Phosphorus - 21 mg Calcium - 13 mg Iron - 0.14 mg Magnesium - 7 mg Sodium - 2 mg Zinc - 0.13 mg Copper - 0.04 mg Manganese - 0.092 mg Selenium - 0.4 mcg Also contains small amounts other minerals.	Vitamin C - 3.1 mg Niacin - 0.099 mg Vitamin B1 (thiamine) - 0.025 mg Vitamin B2 (riboflavin) - 0.014 mg Vitamin B6 - 0.077 mg Pantothenic Acid - 0.068 mg

			Folate - 9 mcg Vitamin A - 1 IU Vitamin K - 0.3 mcg Vitamin E - 0.01 mg Contains some other vitamins in small amounts.
Parsnip	One cup of parsnip, cooked, boiled, drained, with no added salt has 2.06 grams protein, 111 calories and 5.6 grams of dietary fiber.	Potassium - 573 mg Phosphorus - 108 mg Magnesium - 45 mg Calcium - 58 mg Iron - 0.9 mg Sodium - 16 mg Zinc - 0.41 mg Copper - 0.215 mg Manganese - 0.459 mg Selenium - 2.7 mcg Also contains small amounts of other minerals.	Vitamin C - 20.3 mg Niacin - 1.129 mg Vitamin B1 (thiamine) - 0.129 mg Vitamin B2 (riboflavin) - 0.08 mg Vitamin B6 - 0.145 mg Folate - 90 mcg Pantothenic Acid - 0.917 mg Vitamin K - 1.6 mcg Vitamin E - 1.56 mg Contains some other vitamins in small amounts.
Peas	One cup of boiled peas with no salt added contains 8.58 grams of protein, 134 calories and 8.8 grams of fiber.	Potassium - 434 mg Phosphorus - 187 mg Magnesium - 62 mg Calcium - 43 mg Sodium - 5 mg Selenium - 3.0 mg Iron - 2.46 mg Zinc - 1.9 mg Manganese - 0.84 mg Copper - 0.277 mg Also contains small amounts of other minerals.	Vitamin A - 1282 IU Vitamin C - 22.7 mg Niacin - 3.234 mg Folate - 101 mcg Vitamin B1 (thiamine) - 0.414 mg Vitamin B2 (riboflavin) - 0.238 mg Vitamin B6 - 0.346 mg Pantothenic Acid - 0.245 mg Vitamin K - 41.4 mcg Vitamin E - 0.22 mg Contains some other vitamins in small

			amounts.
Potatoes	One medium baked potato without salt contains 4.33 grams of protein, 161 calories and 3.8 grams of fiber.	Potassium - 926 mg Phosphorus - 121 mg Magnesium - 48 mg Calcium - 26 mg Iron - 1.87 mg Sodium - 17 mg Zinc - 0.62 mg Copper - 0.204 mg Manganese - 0.379 mg Selenium - 0.7 mcg Also contains small amounts of other minerals.	Vitamin C - 16.6 mg Niacin - 2.439 mg Vitamin B1 (thiamine) - 0.111 mg Vitamin B2 (riboflavin) - 0.083 mg Pantothenic Acid - 0.65 mg Vitamin B6 - 0.538 mg Folate - 48 mcg Vitamin A - 17 IU Vitamin K - 3.5 mcg Vitamin E - 0.07 mg Contains some other vitamins in small amounts.
Pumpkin	One cup of pumpkin, cooked, boiled, drained, with no added salt has 1.76 grams protein, 49 calories and 2.7 grams of dietary fiber.	Potassium - 564 mg Phosphorus - 74 mg Magnesium - 22 mg Calcium - 37 mg Iron - 1.4 mg Sodium - 2 mg Zinc - 0.56 mg Copper - 0.223 mg Manganese - 0.218 mg Selenium - 0.5 mcg Also contains small amounts of other minerals.	Vitamin C - 11.5 mg Niacin - 1.012 mg Vitamin B1 (thiamine) - 0.076 mg Vitamin B2 (riboflavin) - 0.191 mg Vitamin B6 - 0.108 mg Folate - 22 mcg Pantothenic Acid - 0.492 mg Vitamin A - 12230 IU Vitamin K - 2 mcg Vitamin E - 1.96 mg Contains some other vitamins in small amounts.
Radish	One half cup of radishes, raw, has 0.39 grams protein, 9 calories and 0.9 grams of	Potassium - 135 mg Phosphorus - 12 mg Magnesium - 6 mg Calcium - 14 mg Iron - 0.2 mg Sodium - 23 mg	Vitamin C - 8.6 mg Niacin - 0.147 mg Vitamin B1 (thiamine) - 0.007 mg Vitamin

		Zinc - 0.16 mg Copper - 0.029 mg Manganese - 0.04 mg Selenium - 0.3 mcg Also contains small amounts of other minerals.	B2 (riboflavin) - 0.023 mg Vitamin B6 - 0.041 mg Folate - 14 mcg Pantothenic Acid - 0.096 mg Vitamin A - 4 IU Vitamin K - 0.8 mcg Contains some other vitamins in small amounts.
Rapini	One cup of rapini, raw, has 1.27 grams protein, 9 calories and 1.1 grams of dietary fiber.	Potassium - 78 mg Phosphorus - 29 mg Magnesium - 9 mg Calcium - 43 mg Iron - 0.86 mg Sodium - 13 mg Zinc - 0.31 mg Copper - 0.017 mg Manganese - 0.158 mg Selenium - 0.4 mcg Also contains small amounts of other minerals.	Vitamin C - 8.1 mg Niacin - 0.488 mg Vitamin B1 (thiamine) - 0.065 mg Vitamin B2 (riboflavin) - 0.052 mg Vitamin B6 - 0.068 mg Folate - 33 mcg Pantothenic Acid - 0.129 mg Vitamin A - 1049 IU Vitamin K - 89.6 mcg Vitamin E - 0.65 mg Contains some other vitamins in small amounts.
Spinach	One cup of raw spinach contains 0.86 grams of protein, 7 calories and 0.7 grams of fiber.	Potassium - 167 mg Phosphorus - 15 mg Magnesium - 24 mg Calcium - 30 mg Iron - 0.81 mg Sodium - 24 mg Zinc - 0.16 mg Copper - 0.039 mg Manganese - 0.269 mg Selenium - 0.3 mcg Also contains small amounts of other minerals.	Vitamin C - 8.4 mg Niacin - 0.217 mg Vitamin B1 (thiamine) - 0.023 mg Vitamin B2 (riboflavin) - 0.057 mg Vitamin B6 - 0.059 mg Pantothenic Acid - 0.02 mg Folate - 58 mcg Vitamin A - 2813 mg Vitamin K - 144.9 mcg

			Vitamin E - 0.61 mg Contains some other vitamins in small amounts.
Spirulina (seaweed) 	One cup of dried spirulina has 64.37 grams protein, 325 calories and 4 grams of dietary fiber.	Potassium - 1527 mg Phosphorus - 132 mg Magnesium - 218 mg Calcium - 134 mg Iron - 31.92 mg Zinc - 2.24 mg Manganese - 2.128 mg Sodium - 1174 mg Selenium - 8.1 mg Copper - 6.832 mg Also contains small amounts of other minerals.	Vitamin C - 11.3 mg Niacin - 14.358 mg Vitamin B1 (thiamine) - 2.666 mg Vitamin B2 (riboflavin) - 4.11 mg Vitamin B6 - 0.408 mg Pantothenic Acid - 3.898 mg Folate - 105 mcg Vitamin A - 638 mg Vitamin K - 28.6 mcg Vitamin E - 5.6 mg Contains some other vitamins in small amounts.
Spaghetti squash 	One cup of spaghetti squash, cooked, boiled, drained, and with no added salt contains 1.02 grams protein, 42 calories and 2.2 grams of dietary fiber.	Potassium - 181 mg Phosphorus - 22 mg Magnesium - 17 mg Calcium - 33 mg Iron - 0.53 mg Sodium - 28 mg Zinc - 0.31 mg Copper - 0.054 mg Manganese - 0.169 mg Selenium - 0.5 mcg Also contains small amounts of other minerals.	Vitamin C - 5.4 mg Niacin - 1.256 mg Vitamin B1 (thiamine) - 0.059 mg Vitamin B2 (riboflavin) - 0.034 mg Vitamin B6 - 0.153 mg Pantothenic Acid - 0.55 mg Folate - 12 mcg Vitamin A - 170 mg Vitamin K - 1.2 mcg Vitamin E - 0.19 mg Contains some other vitamins in small amounts.
Squash, Summer	One cup of sliced summer squash,	Potassium - 319 mg Phosphorus - 52 mg	Vitamin C - 20.9 mg

	boiled with no added salt contains 1.87 grams of protein, 41 calories and 2 grams of fiber.	Magnesium - 29 mg Calcium - 40 mg Sodium - 2 mg Iron - 0.67 mg Manganese - 0.283 mg Selenium - 0.4 mg Zinc - 0.4 mg Copper - 0.117 mg Also contains small amounts of other minerals.	Niacin - .913 mg Vitamin B1 (thiamine) - 0.077 mg Vitamin B2 (riboflavin) - 0.045 mg Vitamin B6 - 0.14 mg Pantothenic Acid - 0.581 mg Folate - 41 mcg Vitamin A - 2011 mg Vitamin K - 7.9 mcg Vitamin E - 0.22 mg Contains some other vitamins in small amounts.
Squash, Winter 	One cup of cubed winter squash, baked with no added salt contains 1.82 grams of protein, 76 calories and 5.7 grams of fiber.	Potassium - 494 mg Phosphorus - 39 mg Magnesium - 27 mg Calcium - 45 mg Sodium - 2 mg Iron - 0.9 mg Zinc - 0.45 mg Copper - 0.168 mg Manganese - 0.383 mg Selenium - 0.8 mcg Also contains small amounts of other minerals.	Vitamin C - 19.7 mg Niacin - 1.015 mg Vitamin B1 (thiamine) - 0.033 mg Vitamin B2 (riboflavin) - 0.137 mg Vitamin B6 - 0.33 mg Folate - 41 mcg Pantothenic Acid - 0.48 mg Vitamin A - 10707 mg Vitamin K - 9 mcg Vitamin E - 0.25 mg Contains some other vitamins in small amounts.
Sweet Potatoes 	One medium sweet potato baked in its skin contains 2.29 grams of protein, 103 calories and 3.8 grams of fiber.	Potassium - 542 mg Phosphorus - 62 mg Magnesium - 31 mg Calcium - 43 mg Sodium - 41 mg Iron - 0.79 mg Selenium - 0.2 mg Manganese - 0.567 mg Zinc - 0.36 mg	Vitamin C - 22.3 mg Niacin - 1.695 mg Vitamin B1 (thiamine) - 0.122 mg Vitamin B2 (riboflavin) - 0.121 mg

		Copper - 0.184 mg Also contains small amounts of other minerals.	Vitamin B6 - 0.326 mg Pantothenic Acid - 1.008 mg Folate - 7 mcg Vitamin A - 21,909 mg Vitamin K - 2.6 mcg Vitamin E - 0.81 mg Contains some other vitamins in small amounts.
Swiss chard 	One cup of Swiss chard, cooked, boiled, drained, has 3.29 grams protein, 35 calories and 3.7 grams of dietary fiber.	Potassium - 961 mg Phosphorus - 58 mg Magnesium - 150 mg Calcium - 102 mg Iron - 3.95 mg Sodium - 313 mg Zinc - 0.58 mg Copper - 0.285 mg Manganese - 0.585 mg Selenium - 1.6 mcg Also contains small amounts of other minerals.	Vitamin C - 31.5 mg Niacin - 0.63 mg Vitamin B1 (thiamine) - 0.06 mg Vitamin B2 (riboflavin) - 0.15 mg Vitamin B6 - 0.149 mg Pantothenic Acid - 0.285 mg Folate - 16 mcg Vitamin A - 10717 IU Vitamin K - 572.8 mcg Vitamin E - 3.31 mg Contains some other vitamins in small amounts.
Taro 	One cup of taro, raw, has 1.56 grams protein, 116 calories and 4.3 grams of dietary fiber.	Potassium - 615 mg Phosphorus - 87 mg Magnesium - 34 mg Calcium - 45 mg Iron - 0.57 mg Sodium - 11 mg Zinc - 0.24 mg Copper - 0.179 mg Manganese - 0.398 mg Selenium - 0.7 mcg Also contains small amounts of other minerals.	Vitamin C - 4.7 mg Niacin - 0.624 mg Vitamin B1 (thiamine) - 0.099 mg Vitamin B2 (riboflavin) - 0.026 mg Vitamin B6 - 0.294 mg Folate - 23 mcg Pantothenic Acid - 0.315 mg Vitamin A - 79 IU Vitamin K - 1 mcg

			Vitamin E - 2.48 mg Contains some other vitamins in small amounts.
Turnip 	One cup of turnips, boiled with no added salt, has 1.11 grams protein, 34 calories and 3.1 grams of dietary fiber.	Potassium - 276 mg Phosphorus - 41 mg Magnesium - 14 mg Calcium - 51 mg Iron - 0.28 mg Zinc - 0.19 mg Copper - 0.003 mg Manganese - 0.111 mg Selenium - 0.3 mcg Also contains small amounts other minerals.	Vitamin C - 18.1 mg Niacin - 0.466 mg Vitamin B1 (thiamine) - 0.042 mg Vitamin B2 (riboflavin) - 0.036 mg Vitamin B6 - 0.105 mg Pantothenic Acid - 0.222 mg Folate - 14 mcg Vitamin K - 0.2 mcg Vitamin E - 0.03 mg Contains some other vitamins in small amounts.
Yellow squash 	One cup of yellow (crookneck) squash, raw, has 1.28 grams protein, 24 calories and 1.3 grams of dietary fiber.	Potassium - 282 mg Phosphorus - 41 mg Magnesium - 25 mg Calcium - 27 mg Iron - 0.56 mg Sodium - 3 mg Zinc - 0.37 mg Copper - 0.117 mg Manganese - 0.218 mg Selenium - 0.3 mcg Also contains small amounts of other minerals.	Vitamin C - 24.5 mg Niacin - 0.569 mg Vitamin B1 (thiamine) - 0.065 mg Vitamin B2 (riboflavin) - 0.052 mg Vitamin B6 - 0.132 mg Folate - 24 mcg Pantothenic Acid - 0.203 mg Vitamin A - 190 IU Vitamin K - 4.1 mcg Vitamin E - 0.17 mg Contains some other vitamins in small amounts.

You can see from the table above that there is a large variety of vegetables available for you to eat and enjoy! At the same time all these vegetables will provide a continuous alkalizing and healing effect in different degrees.

Let us now take a more detailed look at the key minerals and vitamins contained in the foods that help your body achieve its natural level of alkalinity:

Alkalizing and cancer preventative MINERALS, ANTIOXIDANT VITAMINS and foods rich in them:

ALKALIZING MINERALS

Potassium: pH 14
Cesium: pH 14
Calcium: pH 12
Magnesium: pH 9
Selenium: pH 9
Sodium: pH 14
Rubidium: pH 14

ANTIOXIDANT VITAMINS

Vitamin A and the Carotenoids

Vitamin A carotenoids are found naturally in fruits and vegetables, which are yellow, red and green. This antioxidant family includes alpha-carotene, beta-carotene, lycopene, lutein and zeaxanthin. Working as **anti-cancer agents**, carotenoids decrease the risk of cataracts and age-related macular degeneration as well as helping to inhibit

56

heart disease. The body converts carotenoid energy into vitamin A and reduces the oxidation of DNA.

Vitamin C

Vitamin C works in conjunction with vitamin E to maintain its potency. Due to its water solubility, vitamin C works in bodily fluids as an effective free-radical scavenger. According to the book "Prescription for Nutritional Healing" by Dr. Phyllis A. Balch, the cells of the brain and spinal cord can be protected by significant amounts of vitamin C. This powerful antioxidant also guards against atherosclerosis by preventing free radical damage to the artery walls.

Vitamin E

Useful for preventing the oxidation of fats, vitamin E prevents the cell's protective coatings from becoming rancid due to the **oxidation** of **free radicals**. Vitamin E is fat-soluble. It enhances the **immune response**, helps prevent cataracts and decreases the risk for coronary artery disease. In order for the body to maintain adequate levels of vitamin E, the antioxidant zinc must also be present.

Selenium

An essential trace mineral, selenium works with vitamin E to protect cell membranes and tissues. Selenium works by targeting natural hydrogen peroxide in the body and converting it into water. Found naturally in **asparagus**, **garlic** and **grains**, selenium helps guard the heart, liver and lungs against **free radical** damage.

Coenzyme Q10

Though coenzyme Q10 is not technically a vitamin, it is produced naturally in the body and levels often decrease with age. Found in highest concentrations in the heart and liver, coenzyme Q10 plays a crucial role in the **generation** of proper **cellular energy**. Working in the **mitochondria** of the cell, coenzyme Q10 helps to metabolize carbohydrates and fats and has a natural anti-aging effect. Supplementing the diet with coenzyme Q10 may be especially beneficial for heart patients, as it is known to increase circulation and stimulate the **immune system.**

Alpha-Lipoic Acid

Working as a "recycler" of vitamins C and E, alpha-lipoic acid restores the antioxidant properties of vitamins after they have **neutralized free radicals** in the body. Stimulating the absorption of other vitamins, alpha-lipoic acid is especially beneficial for **detoxifying the liver** of metal pollutants and lowering blood cholesterol levels.

Having read all this information that I've laid out for you, you **don't have to rush to a shop** and buy minerals and vitamins in tablet form; our body digests and works best with minerals and vitamins - and you get the most benefit from them - when they are taken into the body as **whole foods** like the organic **vegetables**, **fruits** and other foods you will become familiar with from the charts contained in my book.

JUICING

*"To **improve** is to **change**; to **be perfect** is **to change** often."*

Winston Churchill

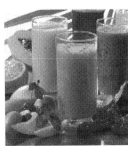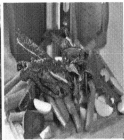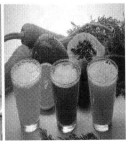

I want you to enjoy your more alkaline diet so here are several of my favorite combinations of the Super Alkaline Fresh Vegetables and Fresh Fruit Juices for You to enjoy and which will rebuild your body's natural defensive capabilities:

You do not have to go to a juice bar – you can also start making and drinking **fresh juices from organic fruits and vegetables** in your own kitchen and play with the ingredients according to your **own taste preferences**. I can give you a few ideas for **fresh juice** recipes and then you can involve your own creativity and imagination and create your own recipes knowing which vegetables and fruits to use from the charts in my book.

Sample these Delicious Fresh Vegetable Juice mixes – try to confirm from **organic sources**:

1. Apple
   Carrot
   Celery
   Ginger
   Spinach
   Chia Seeds (or as a powder to have the best absorption)
   Fresh Wheatgrass - SUPER ALKALINE
   (You can use wheatgrass powder or order frozen wheatgrass if fresh wheatgrass juice is not accessible.)

2. Kale
   Cucumber
   Garlic
   Alfalfa
   Celeriac
   Chia Seeds as a powder
   Fresh Wheatgrass - SUPER ALKALINE

3. Apple - chew the seeds
   Pumpkin
   Spirulina
   Ginseng
   Chia Seeds as a powder
   Fresh Wheatgrass - SUPER ALKALINE

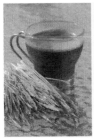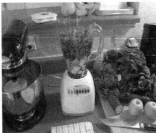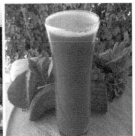

4. Alfalfa grass
   Spirulina
   Brussels sprouts
   Broccoli
   Chia Seeds as a powder
   Fresh Wheatgrass - SUPER ALKALINE

5. Kale
   Carrots
   Apricot seeds (kernels) – 2-3 pieces
   Alfalfa
   Bamboo
   Chia Seeds as a powder
   Fresh Wheatgrass - SUPER ALKALINE

Please experiment with the ingredients and amounts to find the combination that you like! You have to enjoy the taste. Please feel free to play with quantities according to your personal taste and preferences

Now let's look at a few fresh **fruits - organic sources**:

1. Papaya
   Mango
   Lime
   Blackberries
   Chia Seeds as a powder
   Fresh Wheatgrass - SUPER ALKALINE

2. Banana
   Papaya
   Coconut
   Apple
   Chia Seeds as a powder
   Fresh Wheatgrass - SUPER ALKALINE

3. Pomegranate
   Mango
   Cranberry
   Papaya
   Chia Seeds as a powder
   Fresh Wheatgrass - SUPER ALKALINE

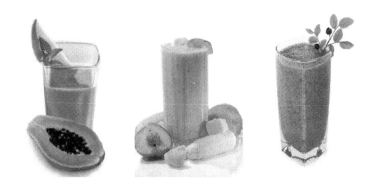

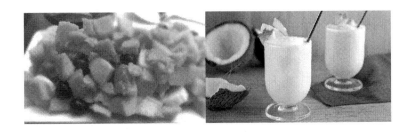

Chapter 3

What your blood cells wish they could tell you about Mitochondria, the Brain and Foods we consume

*The reason people find it **so hard to be happy** is that they always see the past better than it was, the **present worse than it is**, and the future less resolved **than it will be** –*

Marcel Pagnol.

To help the body with **growing new cells** and **strengthening existing cells**, we need to understand the vital part played by Mitochondria.

Mitochondria, which are tiny structures inside our cells, are the powerhouse of our cells.

Mitochondria are the biological engines that convert **carbohydrates**, **proteins** and **fats** into the energy consumed by the entire body. **Efficient mitochondria** provide the **energy** for our **cells** and keep our cells **healthy**. Healthy cells are the **key** to a whole range of benefits for our brain and body, including increased energy levels.

"The main function of the mitochondrion is the production of energy, in the form of adenosine triphosphate (ATP). The cell uses this energy to perform the specific work necessary for cell survival and function.

*The raw materials used to generate ATP are the **foods** that we eat, or tissues within the body that are broken down in a process called catabolism. The breaking down of food into simpler molecules such as **carbohydrates, fats**, and **protein** is called **metabolism**. These molecules are then transferred into the **mitochondria**, where further processing occurs. The reactions within the mitochondria produce specific molecules that can have their electrical charges separated within the inner mitochondrial membrane. These charged molecules are processed within the five electron transport chain complexes to finally combine with oxygen to make ATP. The process of the charged substances combining with oxygen is called **oxidation**, while the chemical reaction making ATP is called phosphorylation. The overall process is called oxidative phosphorylation. The product produced by this process is ATP.*

*Cell death can occur either by injury due to **toxic exposure**, by mechanical damage, or by an orderly process called **programmed cell death** or **apoptosis**. Programmed cell death occurs during development as the organism is pruning away unwanted, excess cells. It also occurs during infections with viruses, **cancer therapy**, or in the **immune response to illness**. The process of programmed cell death is another function of **mitochondria**.*

Normally, ATP production is coupled to oxygen consumption. During abnormal states such as fever, **cancer**, or **stroke**, or when dysfunction occurs within the mitochondria, more oxygen is consumed or **required** than is actually used to make ATP. The mitochondria become partially "uncoupled" and produce **highly reactive oxygen species called free radicals.** When the production of free radicals overwhelms the mitochondria's ability to **"detoxify"** them, the excess free radicals damage mitochondrial function by changing the **mitochondrial DNA**, proteins, and membranes. As this process continues, it can induce the cell to undergo **apoptosis**. Abnormal cell death due to mitochondrial dysfunction can interfere with organ function.

Mitochondria are involved in **building**, **breaking down**, and **recycling products** needed for **proper cell functioning**. For example, some of the building blocks of DNA and RNA occur within the mitochondria. Mitochondria are also involved in making parts of blood and hormones such as **estrogen** and **testosterone**. They are required for **cholesterol metabolism**, **neurotransmitter metabolism, and detoxification** of ammonia in the urea cycle. **Thus, if mitochondria do not function properly, not only energy production but also cell-specific products needed for normal cell functioning will be affected.**" By Russell P. Saneto, D.O., Ph.D., Children's Hospital and Regional Medical Center/University of Washington School of Medicine, Seattle, WA.

Mitochondria were first proposed to be relevant to cancer by Nobel prize-winner Dr Otto Warburg who reported that cancer cells exhibited "aerobic-glycolysis". Although this was originally interpreted as indicating that the function of mitochondria was defective, we now understand that cancer cells are in an altered metabolic state.

From the information you have read above, you can appreciate the **crucial importance** of the **quality of the food** we are providing to our bodies to achieve good health, the overall quality of our life and the quality of our brain power and energy levels we experience every day. Giving good quality nutritional material for our cells to work with (food that we consume every day) will give our cells the opportunity to do their job properly. You only have to provide the material and they will do an excellent job for you! Our body is such an intelligent factory, requiring very **high quality materials** in order to produce very **high quality results**!

Mitochondria are probably the most important structures found in cells. They make up as much as 60% of the volume of muscle cells and 40% of the volume of **heart cells**. They are involved in almost every energy intensive process in the cell and many diseases that deal with energy balances (**diabetes, sarcopenia, cancer, multiple sclerosis**) can be traced back to defects in a cell's mitochondria. In fact, mitochondria are so important to the survival of the cell that they even contain their own DNA so they don't have to depend on the nucleus to repair or replace themselves.

Here is the extraordinary story of Professor of Medicine Dr. Terry Wahls MD who was diagnosed with Multiple Sclerosis.

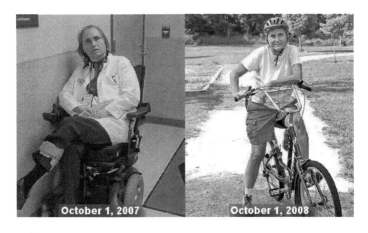

As you will read, Dr. Terry Wahls decided to pay attention to the important role **mitochondria plays in our overall health** and actually cured herself by changing her nutrition much the same way that you will be changing yours. Her main shift was a change in her daily diet. She included lots of green organic vegetables (**alkalizing**) that you saw in the chart above, **grass-fed meat** (you can have fish, preferably local catch or any wild fish available at your local supermarket, ideally not more than a couple of times a week). She also avoided **foods that contain too much acidity**.

Here is Dr. Terry Wahl's story in her own words:

"...I am a clinical professor of medicine at the University of Iowa Carver College of Medicine in Iowa City, Iowa, U.S.A., where I teach internal medicine residents in their primary care clinics. I also do clinical research and have published over 60 peer-reviewed scientific abstracts, posters and papers.

In addition to being a doctor, I am also a patient with a chronic, progressive disease. I was diagnosed with relapsing remitting multiple sclerosis in 2000, just as I began working for the University. By 2003 I had transitioned to secondary progressive multiple sclerosis. I underwent chemotherapy in an attempt to slow the disease and began using a tilt-recline wheelchair because of weakness in my back muscles. It was clear: eventually I would become bedridden by my disease. I wanted to forestall that fate as long as possible.

Because of my academic medical training, I know that research in animal models of disease is often 20 or 30 years ahead of clinical practice. Hoping to find something to arrest my descent into becoming bedridden, I used PubMed.gov to begin searching the scientific articles about the latest multiple sclerosis research. Night after night, I relearned biochemistry, cellular physiology, and neuroimmunology to understand the articles. Unfortunately, most of the studies were testing drugs that were years away from FDA approval. Then it occurred to me to search for vitamins and supplements that helped any kind of progressive brain disorder. Slowly I created a list of nutrients important to brain health and began taking them as supplements. The steepness of my decline slowed, for which I was grateful, but I still was declining.

In the fall of 2007, I had an important epiphany. What if I redesigned my diet so that I was getting those important brain nutrients not from supplements but from the foods I ate? It took more time to create this new diet, intensive directed nutrition, which I designed to provide optimal nutrition for my brain. At that time, I also learned about neuromuscular electrical stimulation and convinced my physical therapist to give me a test session. It hurt, a lot, but I also felt euphoric when it was finished, likely because of the endorphins my body released in response to the electrical stimulation. In December 2007, I began my intensive directed nutrition along with a program of progressive exercise, electrical stimulation, and daily meditation. The results stunned my physician, my family and me: within a year, I was able to walk through the hospital without a cane and even complete an 18-mile bicycle tour.

In 2007 I was losing my phone and keys and was afraid my chief of staff would soon be calling me to his office to tell me that it was time to revoke my clinical privileges. I expected to become ever more dependent because of my illness. Instead, within a year of starting my regimen I regained the ability to commute to work on my bicycle, do my rounds on foot without canes or wheelchairs, conduct clinical trials and write grants, all by making changes to the foods I ate and keeping up with exercise and stress management…"

Thanks to Dr. Terry Wahls's own research, knowledge and decision to fight and win the disease and get healthy, she was able in **one year** to exchange a **wheel chair** for a **bicycle** and even enjoy **horse riding**. How many stories like that have you heard?

If she was able to do this you CAN do it as well! You are clearly motivated to make the decision to make some changes to your diet and to say NO to a few things you probably liked to eat very much in your past and replace them with more healthy options that you already learned, that are available from the earlier tables I shared with you.

God gave us such a wonderful gift – the gift of choice…so what is your choice now? Take a few minutes, sit very quietly and try to look inside your beautiful soul and decide what your **choice is now for your body**?

You understand now that you **can** fight and beat cancer disease because you know how to create an alkaline body environment that prevents cancer cells from surviving and being active. So it is time to make that choice and use your mind and will power to create a "super microclimate" in your body for your healthy cells to have as much cancer neutralizing nutrition as you can give them. **You have no idea how much your cells will pay you in return.** Just provide for them the necessary environment to function at

71

their best. Our body was designed by a very intelligent source; depending on **what** and **how much** you decide to help it, it can **destroy** itself or it can **heal** itself!

We've fully covered vegetables that would be very helpful for your system in the vegetable chart in an earlier chapter and you probably also interested in the full list of fruits that are helpful to eat or make juices from... Here they are for you! All fruits shown below should be ripe and grown organically.

Best Alkalizing Fruits with Mineral and Vitamin content

Fruits	Amount	Minerals Contained	Vitamins Contained
Apple	One medium apple with skin contains 0.47 grams of protein, 95 calories, and 4.4 grams of dietary fiber.	Potassium - 195 mg Calcium - 11 mg Phosphorus - 20 mg Magnesium - 9 mg Manganese - 0.064 mg Iron - 0.22 mg Sodium - 2 mg Copper - 0.049 mg Zinc - 0.07 mg Also contains a trace amount of other minerals.	Vitamin A - 98 IU Vitamin B1 (thiamine) - 0.031 mg Vitamin B2 (riboflavin) - 0.047 mg Niacin - 0.166 mg Folate - 5 mcg Pantothenic Acid - 0.111 mg Vitamin B6 - 0.075 mg Vitamin C - 8.4 mg Vitamin E - 0.33 mg Vitamin K - 4 mcg Contains some other vitamins in small amounts.
Avocado	One medium avocado contains 4.02 grams of	Potassium - 975 mg Phosphorus - 105 mg Magnesium - 58 mg Calcium - 24 mg	Vitamin A - 293 IU Vitamin C - 20.1 mg Vitamin B1 (thiamine) - 0.135 mg

	protein, 322 calories and 13.5 grams of fiber.	Sodium - 14 mg Iron - 1.11 mg Selenium 0.8 mcg Manganese - 0.285 mg Copper - 0.382 mg Zinc - 1.29 mg Also contains small amounts of other minerals.	Vitamin B2 (riboflavin) - 0.261 mg Niacin - 3.493 mg Folate - 163 mcg Pantothenic Acid - 2.792 mg Vitamin B6 - .517 mg Vitamin E - 4.16 mg Vitamin K - 42.2 mcg Contains some other vitamins in small amounts.
Banana	One medium banana contains 1.29 grams of protein, 105 calories and 3.1 grams of dietary fiber.	Potassium - 422 mg Phosphorus - 26 mg Magnesium - 32 mg Calcium - 6 mg Sodium - 1 mg Iron - 0.31 mg Selenium 1.2 mcg Manganese - 0.319 mg Copper - 0.092 mg Zinc - 0.18 mg Also contains small amounts of other minerals.	Vitamin A - 76 IU Vitamin B1 (thiamine) - 0.037 mg Vitamin B2 (riboflavin) - 0.086 mg Niacin - 0.785 mg Folate - 24 mcg Pantothenic Acid - 0.394 mg Vitamin B6 - 0.433 mg Vitamin C - 10.3 mg Vitamin E - 0.12 mg Vitamin K - 0.6 mcg Contains some other vitamins in small amounts.
Blackberries	One cup of blackberries contains 2 grams of protein, 62 calories and 7.6 grams of dietary fiber.	Potassium - 233 mg Phosphorus - 32 mg Magnesium - 29 mg Calcium - 42 mg Sodium - 1 mg Iron - 0.89 mg Selenium 0.6 mcg Manganese - 0.93 mg Copper - 0.238 mg Zinc - 0.76 mg Also contains small amounts of other minerals.	Vitamin A - 308 IU Vitamin B1 (thiamine) - 0.029 mg Vitamin B2 (riboflavin) - 0.037 mg Niacin - 0.93 mg Folate - 36 mcg Pantothenic Acid - 0.397 mg Vitamin B6 - 0.043 mg Vitamin C - 30.2 mg Vitamin E - 1.68 mg Vitamin K - 28.5 mcg Contains some other vitamins in small amounts.
Blackcurrants	One cup of blackcurrants contains 1.57 grams of protein and 71 calories.	Potassium - 361 mg Phosphorus - 66 mg Magnesium - 27 mg Calcium - 62 mg Sodium - 2 mg Iron - 1.72 mg Manganese - 0.287 mg Copper - 0.096 mg Zinc - 0.3 mg Also contains small amounts of	Vitamin A - 258 IU Vitamin B1 (thiamine) - 0.056 mg Vitamin B2 (riboflavin) - 0.056 mg Niacin - 0.336 mg Pantothenic Acid - 0.446 mg Vitamin B6 - 0.074 mg Vitamin C - 202.7 mg

		other minerals.	Vitamin E - 1.12 mg Contains some other vitamins in small amounts.
Blueberries	One cup of blueberries contains 1.1 grams of protein, 84 calories and 3.6 grams of dietary fiber.	Potassium - 114 mg Phosphorus - 18 mg Magnesium - 9 mg Calcium - 9 mg Sodium - 1 mg Iron - 0.41 mg Selenium 0.1 mcg Manganese - 0.497 mg Zinc - 0.24 mg Also contains small amounts of other minerals.	Vitamin A - 217 IU Vitamin B1 (thiamine) - 0.055 mg Vitamin B2 (riboflavin) - 0.061 mg Niacin - 0.08 mg Folate - 9 mcg Pantothenic Acid - 0.184 mg Vitamin B6 - 0.077 mg Vitamin C - 14.4 mg Vitamin E - 2.29 mg Vitamin K - 28.6 mcg Contains some other vitamins in small amounts.
Boysenberries	One cup of frozen boysenberries contains 1.45 grams of protein, 66 calories and 7 grams of dietary fiber.	Potassium - 183 mg Phosphorus - 36 mg Magnesium - 21 mg Calcium - 36 mg Sodium - 1 mg Iron - 1.12 mg Selenium 0.3 mcg Manganese - 0.722 mg Copper - 0.106 mg Zinc - 0.29 mg Also contains small amounts of other minerals.	Vitamin A - 88 IU Vitamin B1 (thiamine) - 0.07 mg Vitamin B2 (riboflavin) - 0.049 mg Niacin - 1.012 mg Folate - 83 mcg Pantothenic Acid - 0.33 mg Vitamin B6 - 0.074 mg Vitamin C - 4.1 mg Vitamin E - 1.15 mg Vitamin K - 10.3 mcg Contains some other vitamins in small amounts.
Breadfruit	One cup of fresh breadfruit contains 2.35 grams of protein, 227 calories and 10.8 grams of dietary fiber.	Potassium - 1078 mg Phosphorus - 66 mg Magnesium - 55 mg Calcium - 37 mg Sodium - 4 mg Iron - 1.19 mg Selenium 1.3 mcg Manganese - 0.132 mg Copper - 0.185 mg Zinc - 0.26 mg Also contains small amounts of other minerals.	Vitamin B1 (thiamine) - 0.242 mg Vitamin B2 (riboflavin) - 0.066 mg Niacin - 1.98 mg Folate - 31 mcg Pantothenic Acid - 1.05 mg Vitamin B6 - 0.22 mg Vitamin C - 63.8 mg Vitamin E - 0.22 mg Vitamin K - 1.1 mcg Contains some other vitamins in small amounts.
Cantaloupe	One medium wedge (slice) of	Potassium - 184 mg Phosphorus - 10 mg	Vitamin A - 2334 IU Vitamin B1 (thiamine) -

	cantaloupe contains 0.58 grams of protein, 23 calories and 0.6 grams of dietary fiber.	Magnesium - 8 mg Calcium - 6 mg Sodium - 11 mg Iron - 0.14 mg Selenium 0.3 mcg Manganese - 0.028 mg Copper - 0.028 mg Zinc - 0.12 mg Also contains small amounts of other minerals.	0.028 mg Vitamin B2 (riboflavin) - 0.013 mg Niacin - 0.506 mg Folate - 14 mcg Pantothenic Acid - 0.072 mg Vitamin B6 - 0.05 mg Vitamin C - 25.3 mg Vitamin E - 0.03 mg Vitamin K - 1.7 mcg Contains some other vitamins in small amounts.
Cherimoya 	One cup of diced, fresh cherimoya contains 2.51 grams of protein, 120 calories and 4.8 grams of dietary fiber.	Potassium - 459 mg Phosphorus - 42 mg Magnesium - 27 mg Calcium - 16 mg Sodium - 11 mg Iron - 0.43 mg Manganese - 0.149 mg Copper - 0.11 mg Zinc - 0.26 mg Also contains small amounts of other minerals.	Vitamin B1 (thiamine) - 0.162 mg Vitamin B2 (riboflavin) - 0.21 mg Niacin - 1.03 mg Folate - 37 mcg Pantothenic Acid - 0.552 mg Vitamin B6 - 0.411 mg Vitamin C - 20.2 mg Vitamin A - 8 IU Vitamin E - 0.43 mg Contains some other vitamins in small amounts.
Cherries 	One cup of fresh cherries, with pits, contains 1.46 grams of protein, 87 calories and 2.9 grams of dietary fiber.	Potassium - 306 mg Phosphorus - 29 mg Magnesium - 15 mg Calcium - 18 mg Iron - 0.5 mg Zinc - 0.1 mg Manganese - 0.097 mg Copper - 0.083 mg Also contains small amounts of other minerals.	Vitamin A - 88 IU Vitamin B1 (thiamine) - 0.037 mg Vitamin B2 (riboflavin) - 0.046 mg Niacin - 0.213 mg Folate - 6 mcg Pantothenic Acid - 0.275 mg Vitamin B6 - 0.068 mg Vitamin C - 9.7 mg Vitamin E - 0.1 mg Vitamin K - 2.9 mcg Contains some other vitamins in small amounts.
Chinese pear 	One Chinese (Asian) pear, about 3 inches in diameter, contains 1.38 grams of protein, 116	Potassium - 333 mg Phosphorus - 30 mg Magnesium - 22 mg Calcium - 11 mg Selenium 0.3 mcg Manganese - 0.165 mg Copper - 0.138 mg	Vitamin B1 (thiamine) - 0.025 mg Vitamin B2 (riboflavin) - 0.028 mg Niacin - 0.602 mg Folate - 22 mcg Pantothenic Acid - 0.193

	calories and 9.9 grams of dietary fiber.	Zinc - 0.06 mg Also contains small amounts of other minerals.	mg Vitamin B6 - 0.06 mg Vitamin C - 10.4 mg Vitamin E - 0.33 mg Vitamin K - 12.4 mcg Contains some other vitamins in small amounts.
Cranberries	One cup of cranberries contains 0.39 grams of protein, 46 calories and 4.6 grams of dietary fiber.	Potassium - 85 mg Phosphorus - 13 mg Magnesium - 6 mg Calcium - 8 mg Sodium - 2 mg Iron - 0.25 mg Selenium 0.1 mcg Manganese - 0.36 mg Copper - 0.061 mg Zinc - 0.1 mg Also contains small amounts of other minerals.	Vitamin A - 60 IU Vitamin B1 (thiamine) - 0.012 mg Vitamin B2 (riboflavin) - 0.02 mg Niacin - 0.101 mg Folate - 1 mcg Pantothenic Acid - 0.295 mg Vitamin B6 - 0.057 mg Vitamin C - 13.3 mg Vitamin E - 1.2 mg Vitamin K - 5.1 mcg Contains some other vitamins in small amounts.
Figs	One large, fresh fig contains 0.48 grams of protein, 47 calories and 1.9 grams of dietary fiber.	Potassium - 148 mg Phosphorus - 9 mg Magnesium - 11 mg Calcium - 22 mg Sodium - 1 mg Iron - 0.24 mg Selenium 0.1 mcg Manganese - 0.082 mg Copper - 0.045 mg Zinc - 0.1 mg Also contains small amounts of other minerals.	Vitamin A - 91 IU Vitamin B1 (thiamine) - 0.038 mg Vitamin B2 (riboflavin) - 0.032 mg Niacin - 0.256 mg Folate - 4 mcg Pantothenic Acid - 0.192 mg Vitamin B6 - 0.072 mg Vitamin C - 1.3 mg Vitamin E - 0.07 mg Vitamin K - 3 mcg Contains some other vitamins in small amounts.
Gooseberries	One cup of gooseberries contains 1.32 grams of protein, 66 calories and over 6.5 grams of dietary fiber.	Potassium - 297 mg Phosphorus - 40 mg Magnesium - 15 mg Calcium - 38 mg Sodium - 2 mg Iron - 0.47 mg Selenium 0.9 mcg Manganese - 0.216 mg Copper - 0.105 mg Zinc - 0.18 mg Also contains small amounts of other minerals.	Vitamin A - 435 IU Vitamin B1 (thiamine) - 0.06 mg Vitamin B2 (riboflavin) - 0.045 mg Niacin - 0.45 mg Folate - 9 mcg Pantothenic Acid - 0.429 mg Vitamin B6 - 0.12 mg Vitamin C - 41.5 mg Vitamin E - 0.56 mg Contains some other

			vitamins in small amounts.
Grapes	One cup of grapes contains 1.09 gram of protein, 104 calories and 1.4 grams of dietary fiber.	Potassium - 288 mg Phosphorus - 30 mg Magnesium - 11 mg Calcium - 15 mg Sodium - 3 mg Iron - 0.54 mg Selenium 0.2 mcg Manganese - 0.107 mg Copper - 0.192 mg Zinc - 0.11 mg Also contains small amounts of other minerals.	Vitamin A - 100 IU Vitamin B1 (thiamine) - 0.104 mg Vitamin B2 (riboflavin) - 0.106 mg Niacin - 0.284 mg Folate - 3 mcg Pantothenic Acid - 0.076 mg Vitamin B6 - 0.13 mg Vitamin C - 16.3 mg Vitamin E - 0.29 mg Vitamin K - 22 mcg Contains some other vitamins in small amounts.
Guava	One cup of fresh guava contains 4.21 grams of protein, 112 calories and 8.9 grams of dietary fiber.	Potassium - 688 mg Phosphorus - 66 mg Magnesium - 36 mg Calcium - 30 mg Sodium - 3 mg Iron - 0.43 mg Selenium 1 mcg Manganese - 0.247 mg Copper - 0.38 mg Zinc - 0.38 mg Also contains small amounts of other minerals.	Vitamin A - 1030 IU Vitamin B1 (thiamine) - 0.111 mg Vitamin B2 (riboflavin) - 0.066 mg Niacin - 1.789 mg Folate - 81 mcg Pantothenic Acid - 0.744 mg Vitamin B6 - 0.181 mg Vitamin C - 376.7 mg Vitamin E - 1.2 mg Vitamin K - 4.3 mcg Contains some other vitamins in small amounts.
Lemon	One lemon without peel contains 0.92 grams protein, 24 calories and 2.4 grams of dietary fiber.	Potassium - 116 mg Phosphorus - 13 mg Magnesium - 7 mg Calcium - 22 mg Sodium - 2 mg Iron - 0.5 mg Selenium 0.3 mcg Manganese - 0.025 mg Copper - 0.031 mg Zinc - 0.05 mg Also contains small amounts of other minerals.	Vitamin A - 18 IU Vitamin B1 (thiamine) - 0.034 mg Vitamin B2 (riboflavin) - 0.017 mg Niacin - 0.084 mg Folate - 9 mcg Pantothenic Acid - 0.16 mg Vitamin B6 - 0.067 mg Vitamin C - 44.5 mg Vitamin E - 0.13 mg Contains some other vitamins in small amounts.
Lime	One lime contains 0.47 grams of	Potassium - 68 mg Phosphorus - 12 mg Magnesium - 4 mg	Vitamin A - 34 IU Vitamin B1 (thiamine) - 0.02 mg

	protein, 20 calories and 1.9 grams of dietary fiber.	Calcium - 22 mg Sodium - 1 mg Iron - 0.4 mg Selenium 0.3 mcg Manganese - 0.005 mg Copper - 0.044 mg Zinc - 0.07 mg Also contains small amounts of other minerals.	Vitamin B2 (riboflavin) - 0.013 mg Niacin - 0.134 mg Folate - 5 mcg Pantothenic Acid - 0.145 mg Vitamin B6 - 0.029 mg Vitamin C - 19.5 mg Vitamin E - 0.15 mg Vitamin K - 0.4 mcg Contains some other vitamins in small amounts.
Loganberries 	One cup of frozen loganberries contains 2.23 grams of protein, 81 calories and 7.8 grams of dietary fiber.	Potassium - 213 mg Phosphorus - 38 mg Magnesium - 31 mg Calcium - 38 mg Sodium - 1 mg Iron - 0.94 mg Selenium 0.3 mcg Manganese - 1.833 mg Copper - 0.172 mg Zinc - 0.5 mg Also contains small amounts of other minerals.	Vitamin A - 51 IU Vitamin B1 (thiamine) - 0.074 mg Vitamin B2 (riboflavin) - 0.05 mg Niacin - 1.235 mg Folate - 38 mcg Pantothenic Acid - 0.359 mg Vitamin B6 - 0.096 mg Vitamin C - 22.5 mg Vitamin E - 1.28 mg Vitamin K - 11.5 mcg Contains some other vitamins in small amounts.
Lychee 	One cup of fresh lychees contains 1.58 grams of protein, 125 calories and 2.5 grams of dietary fiber.	Potassium - 325 mg Phosphorus - 59 mg Magnesium - 19 mg Calcium - 10 mg Sodium - 2 mg Iron - 0.59 mg Selenium 1.1 mcg Manganese - 0.104 mg Copper - 0.281 mg Zinc - 0.13 mg Also contains small amounts of other minerals.	Vitamin B1 (thiamine) - 0.021 mg Vitamin B2 (riboflavin) - 0.123 mg Niacin - 1.146 mg Folate - 27 mcg Vitamin B6 - 0.19 mg Vitamin C - 135.8 mg Vitamin E - 0.13 mg Vitamin K - 0.08 mcg Contains some other vitamins in small amounts.
Mango 	One mango without peel contains 1.06 grams of protein, 135 calories and 3.7 grams of dietary fiber.	Potassium - 323 mg Phosphorus - 23 mg Magnesium - 19 mg Calcium - 21 mg Sodium - 4 mg Iron - 0.27 mg Selenium 1.2 mcg Manganese - 0.056 mg Copper - 0.228 mg Zinc - 0.08 mg Also contains small amounts of	Vitamin A - 1584 IU Vitamin B1 (thiamine) - 0.12 mg Vitamin B2 (riboflavin) - 0.118 mg Niacin - 1.209 mg Folate - 29 mcg Pantothenic Acid - 0.331 mg Vitamin B6 - 0.227 mg Vitamin C - 57.3 mg Vitamin E - 2.32 mg

		other minerals.	Vitamin K - 8.7 mcg Contains some other vitamins in small amounts.
Mulberries	One cup of fresh mulberries contains 2.02 grams of protein and 2.4 grams of dietary fiber.	Potassium - 272 mg Phosphorus - 53 mg Magnesium - 25 mg Calcium - 55 mg Sodium - 14 mg Iron - 2.59 mg Selenium 0.8 mcg Copper - 0.084 mg Zinc - 0.17 mg Also contains small amounts of other minerals.	Vitamin A - 35 IU Vitamin B1 (thiamine) - 0.041 mg Vitamin B2 (riboflavin) - 0.141 mg Niacin - 0.868 mg Folate - 8 mcg Vitamin B6 - 0.07 mg Vitamin C - 51 mg Vitamin E - 1.22 mg Vitamin K - 10.9 mcg Contains some other vitamins in small amounts.
Nectarine	One cup of sliced fresh nectarine contains 1.52 grams of protein, 63 calories and 2.4 grams of dietary fiber.	Potassium - 287 mg Phosphorus - 37 mg Magnesium - 13 mg Calcium - 9 mg Iron - 0.4 mg Manganese - 0.077 mg Copper - 0.123 mg Zinc - 0.24 mg Also contains small amounts of other minerals.	Vitamin A - 475 IU Vitamin B1 (thiamine) - 0.049 mg Vitamin B2 (riboflavin) - 0.039 mg Niacin - 1.609 mg Folate - 7 mcg Pantothenic Acid - 0.265 mg Vitamin B6 - 0.036 mg Vitamin C - 7.7 mg Vitamin E - 1.1 mg Vitamin K - 3.1 mcg Contains some other vitamins in small amounts.
Olives	One tablespoon of ripe olives contains 0.07 grams of protein, 10 calories and 0.3 grams of dietary fiber.	Potassium - 1 mg Calcium - 7 mg Sodium - 73 mg Iron - 0.28 mg Selenium 0.1 mcg Manganese - 0.002 mg Copper - 0.021 mg Zinc - 0.02 mg Also contains small amounts of other minerals.	Vitamin A - 34 IU Niacin - 0.003 mg Pantothenic Acid - 0.001 mg Vitamin B6 - 0.001 mg Vitamin C - 0.1 mg Vitamin E - 0.14 mg Vitamin K - 0.1 mcg Contains some other vitamins in small amounts.
Papaya	One cup of cubed fresh papaya contains 0.85 grams of protein, 55 calories and 2.5 grams of dietary fiber.	Potassium - 360 mg Phosphorus - 7 mg Magnesium - 14 mg Calcium - 34 mg Sodium - 4 mg Iron - 0.14 mg Selenium 0.8 mcg Zinc - 0.1 mg	Vitamin A - 1532 IU Vitamin B1 (thiamine) - 0.038 mg Vitamin B2 (riboflavin) - 0.045 mg Niacin - 0.473 mg Folate - 53 mcg Pantothenic Acid - 0.305

		Manganese - 0.015 mg Copper - 0.022 mg Also contains small amounts of other minerals.	mg Vitamin B6 - 0.027 mg Vitamin C - 86.5 mg Vitamin E - 1.02 mg Vitamin K - 3.6 mcg Contains some other vitamins in small amounts.
Passion fruit	One cup of fresh passion fruit contains 5.19 grams of protein, 229 calories and 24.5 grams of dietary fiber.	Potassium - 821 mg Phosphorus - 160 mg Magnesium - 68 mg Calcium - 28 mg Sodium - 66 mg Iron - 3.78 mg Selenium 1.4 mcg Copper - 0.203 mg Zinc - 0.24 mg Also contains small amounts of other minerals.	Vitamin A - 3002 IU Vitamin B2 (riboflavin) - 0.307 mg Niacin - 3.54 mg Folate - 33 mcg Vitamin B6 - 0.236 mg Vitamin C - 70.8 mg Vitamin E - 0.05 mg Vitamin K - 1.7 mcg Contains some other vitamins in small amounts.
Peach	One medium peach (with skin) contains 1.36 grams of protein, 58 calories and 2.2 grams dietary fiber.	Potassium - 285 mg Phosphorus - 30 mg Magnesium - 14 mg Calcium - 9 mg Iron - 0.38 mg Selenium 0.1 mcg Manganese - 0.091 mg Copper - 0.102 mg Zinc - 0.26 mg Also contains small amounts of other minerals.	Vitamin A - 489 IU Vitamin B1 (thiamine) - 0.036 mg Vitamin B2 (riboflavin) - 0.047 mg Niacin - 1.209 mg Folate - 6 mcg Pantothenic Acid - 0.229 mg Vitamin B6 - 0.037 mg Vitamin C - 9.9 mg Vitamin E - 1.09 mg Vitamin K - 3.9 mcg Contains some other vitamins in small amounts.
Pear	One medium pear contains 0.68 grams of protein, 103 calories and 5.5 grams dietary fiber.	Potassium - 212 mg Phosphorus - 20 mg Magnesium - 12 mg Calcium -16 mg Sodium - 2 mg Iron - 0.3 mg Selenium 0.2 mcg Manganese - 0.087 mg Copper - 0.146 mg Zinc - 0.18 mg Also contains small amounts of other minerals.	Vitamin A - 41 IU Vitamin B1 (thiamine) - 0.021 mg Vitamin B2 (riboflavin) - 0.045 mg Niacin - 0.279 mg Folate - 12 mcg Pantothenic Acid - 0.085 mg Vitamin B6 - 0.05 mg Vitamin C - 7.5 mg Vitamin E - 0.21 mg Vitamin K - 8 mcg Contains some other vitamins in small amounts.
Persimmon	One fresh	Potassium - 78 mg	Vitamin C - 16.5 mg

	persimmon contains 0.2 grams of protein and 32 calories.	Phosphorus - 6 mg Calcium - 7 mg Iron - 0.62 mg Also contains small amounts of other minerals.	Contains some other vitamins in small amounts.
Plum 	One cup of sliced, fresh plums contains 1.15 grams of protein, 76 calories and 2.3 grams dietary fiber.	Potassium - 259 mg Phosphorus - 26 mg Magnesium - 12 mg Calcium - 10 mg Iron - 0.28 mg Manganese - 0.086 mg Copper - 0.094 mg Zinc - 0.17 mg Also contains small amounts of other minerals.	Vitamin A - 569 IU Vitamin B1 (thiamine) - 0.046 mg Vitamin B2 (riboflavin) - 0.043 mg Niacin - 0.688 mg Folate - 8 mcg Pantothenic Acid - 0.223 mg Vitamin B6 - 0.048 mg Vitamin C - 15.7 mg Vitamin E - 0.43 mg Vitamin K - 10.6 mcg Contains some other vitamins in small amounts.
Pomegranate 	One fresh pomegranate contains 4.71 grams of protein, 234 calories and 11.3 grams dietary fiber.	Potassium - 666 mg Phosphorus - 102 mg Magnesium - 34 mg Calcium - 28 mg Sodium - 8 mg Iron - 0.85 mg Selenium 1.4 mcg Manganese - 0.336 mg Copper - 0.446 mg Zinc - 0.99 mg Also contains small amounts of other minerals.	Vitamin B1 (thiamine) - 0.189 mg Vitamin B2 (riboflavin) - 0.149 mg Niacin - 0.826 mg Folate - 107 mcg Pantothenic Acid - 1.063 mg Vitamin B6 - 0.211 mg Vitamin C - 28.8 mg Vitamin E - 1.69 mg Vitamin K - 46.2 mcg Contains some other vitamins in small amounts.
Prickly Pear 	One cup of raw prickly pears contains 1.09 grams of protein, 61 calories and 5.4 grams dietary fiber.	Potassium - 328 mg Phosphorus - 36 mg Magnesium - 127 mg Calcium - 83 mg Sodium - 7 mg Iron - 0.45 mg Selenium 0.9 mcg Copper - 0.119 mg Zinc - 0.18 mg Also contains small amounts of other minerals.	Vitamin A - 64 IU Vitamin B1 (thiamine) - 0.021 mg Vitamin B2 (riboflavin) - 0.089 mg Niacin - 0.685 mg Vitamin B6 - 0.089 mg Folate - 9 mcg Vitamin C - 20.9 mg Contains some other vitamins in small amounts.
Star fruit aka	One cup of fresh	Potassium - 176 mg	Vitamin A - 81 IU

Carambola 	star fruit contains 1.37 grams of protein, 41 calories and 3.7 grams dietary fiber.	Phosphorus - 16 mg Magnesium - 13 mg Calcium - 4 mg Sodium - 3 mg Iron - 0.11 mg Selenium 0.8 mcg Manganese - 0.049 mg Copper - 0.181 mg Zinc - 0.16 mg Also contains small amounts of other minerals.	Vitamin B1 (thiamine) - 0.018 mg Vitamin B2 (riboflavin) - 0.021 mg Niacin - 0.484 mg Folate - 16 mcg Pantothenic Acid - 0.516 mg Vitamin B6 - 0.022 mg Vitamin C - 45.4 mg Vitamin E - 0.2 mg Contains some other vitamins in small amounts.
Watermelon 	I medium wedge (slice) of watermelon (about 2 cups edible portion) contains 1.74 grams of protein, 86 calories and 1.1 grams of dietary fiber.	Potassium - 320 mg Phosphorus - 31 mg Magnesium - 29 mg Calcium - 20 mg Sodium - 3 mg Iron - 0.69 mg Selenium 1.1 mcg Manganese - 0.109 mg Copper - 0.12 mg Zinc - 0.29 mg Also contains small amounts of other minerals.	Vitamin A - 1627 IU Vitamin B1 (thiamine) - 0.094 mg Vitamin B2 (riboflavin) - 0.06 mg Niacin - 0.509 mg Folate - 9 mcg Pantothenic Acid - 0.632 mg Vitamin B6 - 0.129 mg Vitamin C - 23.2 mg Vitamin E - 0.14 mg Vitamin K - 0.3 mcg Contains some other vitamins in small amounts.

Chapter 4

What your White Blood Cells want you to know about the COATING on the CANCER CELLS in your body

*"So often we **dwell** on the things that **seem impossible** rather than on the things that **are possible**."*

Marian Wright Edelman

Unfortunately for the body's natural defensive mechanisms, cancer cells are invariably coated with and protected by **mucus and fibrin**. Our goal is to dissolve the coating that will allow our white blood cells army to perform!

Mucus is a glycoprotein (**sugar** and **protein**). **Fibrin** is a **protein** floating in the blood that allows blood to clot. This (biofilm) camouflage of mucus and fibrin prevents the white blood cells of the immune system from **recognizing the cancer cells**. Now you see the connection with why too much meat and animal protein generally in the diet is very dangerous for us. Too much animal protein in the diet as well as refined foods such as **white sugar** and **white flour** deplete pancreatic enzymes (I'll explain in more detail below), as a result helping to open the way for cancer.

Fibrin is also a contributing factor in cardiovascular disease. **Plaque** that builds up on the walls of blood vessels consists of cholesterol, cellular waste, calcium and fibrin. The plaque thickens the vessel wall, while the fibrin and **calcium** harden and cause the wall to lose critical elasticity.

For proper calcium absorption, you need to consume food sources that contain types of calcium that are easily digested, assimilated, and absorbed. It's important to know the special relationship between **magnesium** and **calcium**, as they rely on each other, and **both need** to be present for **proper absorption**. Usually it's in a 2:1 ratio, with two parts calcium to one part of magnesium. One cup of 1-percent low-fat milk provides 305 mg of calcium and 27 mg of magnesium.

As you can see because of the calcium-magnesium ratio in **dairy products**, our bodies **do not properly absorb** the **calcium** it contains. **Excess stores of calcium** accumulate in our **blood** and **urine** as a result can cause kidney problems, formation of kidney stones and gallstones.

A lot of us may or may not know that vegetables, legumes, whole grains, beans, lentils, and nuts contain complete protein, which is different from animal protein. Proteins can be harnessed from many plant sources. Even if you're a vegetarian, you can have alternative protein sources from plant products. The trick is, plant proteins are said to contain almost the same protein value like the ones coming from animals. The advantage is that plants are regarded as excellent sources of vitamins, minerals, fibers and antioxidants that **no animal source can match**.

Common vegetables have protein that you need, and they're complete proteins as well.

According to official sources **we need only 2.5 to 11% of our calories from protein** and common vegetables easily supply that amount. Vegetables average around 22% protein, beans 28%, and grains 13%.

Professional estimates suggest we need as little as 2.5% of our calories from protein. The U.S. government's recommendation is 5-11%, based on various factors.

The World Health Organization recommends a similar amount. And the official recommendations are padded with generous safety margins, to cover people who need more protein than average.

In general, **plant proteins** have **no cholesterol** and fat (saturated fats) as opposed to **animal sources**. That's why if you compare a person who is taking proteins from plants to someone who consumes proteins from animal sources, you can expect the latter to be more likely to develop diseases related to the **heart**, **blood pressure**, etc. and also to be more at risk of increased amounts of **fibrin** floating in the blood that can eventually cover more and more cancer cells making it impossible for white cells to recognize and kill them.

Plant proteins also have more Beta-carotene, dietary fiber, Vitamin C, Vitamin E, folate, Iron, Magnesium and Calcium, etc. as you may have read in the charts above.

As you know, chemotherapy and radiation treatments kill cancer cells in the body as well as some **healthy cells**. We should pay particular attention during these treatments to more sensitive areas of the body like the throat, mouth area and gastro-intestinal tract. Chemotherapy also causes the immune system to overreact and excessive mucus is often the result.

Quiet often one of the side effects of chemotherapy is mucositis.

Mucositis occurs when cancer treatments break down the rapidly divided epithelial cells lining the gastro-intestinal tract, leaving the mucosal tissue open to ulceration and infection. Mucosal tissue, also known as mucosa or the mucous membrane, lines all body passages that communicate with the air, such as the respiratory and alimentary tracts, and have cells and associated glands that secrete **mucus**. The part of this lining that covers the mouth is one of the most sensitive parts of the body and is **particularly vulnerable** to chemotherapy and radiation.

The combination of mucus, excess saliva and pain can make it difficult to eat.

86

To reduce the production of mucus as much as possible please make sure of avoiding any consumption of mucus-producing **dairy products** like milk, cheese, yogurt of any kind, cream and ice cream. This avoidance of dairy products applies to goat dairy products as well.

Dairy products cause the body to produce mucus, especially in the gastro-intestinal tract. **In the human colon**, beta-casomorphin-7 (beta-CM-7), an exorphin derived from the **breakdown of dairy products, stimulates mucus production** from the MUC5AC gene.
This gene has been linked to **mucus hypersecretion** in the pulmonary tracts.

Cow's milk (dairy products - milk, cheese, yogurts of any kind, cream, ice cream and goat products) and fibrin (animal protein like beef, pork etc.) are notoriously the most **cancer-coating foods** we can consume.

Casein, the protein component in milk, is a very thick and coarse substance and is used to make one of the strongest glues known to man. There is **300%** more casein in cows' milk than in human milk.

The **casein** in cows' milk can **clog** and **irritate** the body's **entire respiratory system**. Dairy products are implicated in almost all respiratory problems. Hay fever, asthma, bronchitis, sinusitis, colds, runny noses and ear infections can all be caused by the consumption of dairy products. Dairy products are also the leading cause of allergies.

"There is compelling evidence, now published in top scientific journals and some of which is decades old, showing that cows' milk is associated, possibly even causally, with a wide variety of serious human ailments including various cancers, cardiovascular diseases, diabetes and an array of allergy-related diseases. And, this food contains no nutrients that cannot be better obtained from other far more nutritious and tasty foods." Dr. Colin Campbell

"Inclusion of milk will only reduce your diet's nutritional value and safety. Most of the people on the planet live very healthfully without cow's milk. You can too." Robert M. Kradjian M.D

"I no longer recommend dairy products...there was a time when cow's milk was considered very desirable. But research along with clinical experience has forced doctors and nutritionists to rethink this recommendation" Dr. Benjamin Spock
According to Dr. Julian Whitaker in his 'Health & Healing' newsletter in an article entitled 'Tomorrow's Medicine Today' (October 1998 Vol. 8, No. 10) the notion that milk is healthy for you is "udder" nonsense. While eating fruits,

*vegetables and whole grains has been documented to lower the risk of heart attack, high blood pressure and cancer, the widely touted health benefits of dairy products are questionable at best. In fact, **dairy products** are clearly linked as a **cause** of **osteoporosis, heart disease, obesity, cancer, allergies and diabetes**. He argues that dairy products are anything but "health" foods.*

If you are a big fan of dairy products and love drinking milk by itself or with cereals, I recommend you replace dairy products with very delicious non-dairy alternatives such as **Almond Milk, Brown Rice Milk, Hazelnut Milk, Quinoa Milk, Oat Milk and others made of cereals and nuts. Be careful to avoid any form of Soy Milk.**

Your defensive army of enzymes to kill cancer cells

*"Life is like riding a bicycle. To keep **your balance**, you **must keep moving**."*

Albert Einstein

Now I would like you to understand a connection between low levels of ***enzymes and cancer cells***. Actually doctors in Europe and some doctors in the United States have used enzyme therapy with great results against cancers and literally digested cancer cells.

In the early 1900's Dr. John Beard discovered that pancreatic enzymes destroy cancer cells. Making some brilliant observations, he deduced that cancer cells come from stem cells that become uncontrolled stem cells. He noticed that the fetal pancreas starts working and secreting enzymes at the 56th day of gestation. Fetuses don't digest anything till they are born. Dr. Beard wondered why did the pancreas in the fetus start working so early? He noticed that the day the pancreas started producing enzymes was the day the placenta stopped growing. The enzymes stopped this rapid growth.

His theory about **enzymes and cancer** was that many placental cells remain in our body. When these misplaced placental cells get lost and can start growing, turning cancerous if you don't have enough pancreatic enzymes. (By the way the medical community thought Dr. Beard was crazy. Now a hundred years later, medical science has confirmed the existence of these cells.)

In 1911 Dr Beard tested pancreatic enzymes as cancer prevention in mice and it worked. Unfortunately, he was blackballed by his colleagues and died in obscurity. Decades later Dr. Kelly read about his work, and cured himself of cancer using pancreatic enzymes and started treating and curing many cancer patients using pancreatic enzymes. Dr. Gonzales who has been investigating nutritional approaches to cancer and other degenerative diseases since 1981, and has been in practice in New York

90

since 1987, sent to investigate Dr. Kelly, liked what he saw so much that he also treats cancer using pancreatic enzymes.

In summary, the major reason enzyme levels become depleted in the body is that we eat mostly processed, undernourished, irradiated and cooked food full of sugars and empty carbohydrates like white flour, etc. Big increases of soy food consumption are playing a great role too. We will go much deeper in understanding how soy foods impact our health a bit later. You will be surprised to see how much soy and soybean oil and soy lecithin is sneaked into the food we buy. Unfortunately unless you carefully read the whole list of ingredients - which is usually printed in such small type that a lot of people have difficulty reading it - most of us are unaware that we are eating food products containing soy. I would strongly recommend that you carefully read the list of ingredients of each product you consider buying when doing your food shopping. It's only an investment of time the first time you do it; subsequently you will know what the healthy choices are for you the next time.

Our digestive system was designed to process **raw food**. Raw food, when it is picked **ripe and organic**, has enzymes in it that help break down that food in the upper stomach where it sits for about 30 to 45 minutes. The enzymes in the food predigest that food. Then in the lower stomach the pancreas, when healthy and functioning as it should, excretes more enzymes. Dairy products damage very much the health of the pancreas.

When we eat cooked, undernourished, irradiated and processed foods, most of the enzymes have been killed and the food does not predigest in the upper stomach. So when it reaches the lower stomach *two things happen*. The pancreas must make **extra enzymes** to try and break down the food.

And often food is only partially digested due to poor pancreas function and also to the cold drinks with ice that a lot of people consume these days while eating.

The pancreas, after decades of overworking, eventually is no longer able to produce an adequate supply of enzymes. So you develop **low levels** of all types of enzymes, and your body then *cannot* naturally kill cancer cells using enzymes.

You will be surprised but, in addition, food that is not completely digested all very often makes its way into our bloodstream. This happens especially when people have leaky gut syndrome from **candida** overgrowth. This partially digest food is treated as a toxin, and the immune system has to get rid of it. This puts an additional strain on the already overworked immune system.

Studies have found that the immune system treats the ingestion of cooked food as a toxic poison, causing a jump in white blood cells in an attempt to get rid of it as fast as possible.

"Enzymes dissolve the protein and sugar coating of the cancer cell making it vulnerable to the attack of white blood cells." This has been known since **1905 (Griffin, page 81)**.

*"Fresh **Papaya** is a good source of enzymes. You have the papaya melons as the source of the enzyme Papain. The damasking effect of these enzymes against the pericellular layer of the malignant cell is something very concrete in the immunology of cancer. Now I prefer, rather than advising the use of papaya tablets, that the individual seeking these enzymes get them directly from the fresh papaya fruit. You have nothing to lose by eating fresh papaya melons."* - **Dr. Krebs, Jr.**

Dietary sources of all kinds of enzymes are good, and the consumption of at least 70% fresh foods vs. 30% cooked foods helps **ensure a supply of healthy enzymes** for the body (cooking at temperatures above 116°F destroys enzymes in the food). Fresh foods generally contain all the enzymes required for their own digestion, easing the burden on the digestive system. However, certain foods are more easily digested when cooked because heat breaks down starch (potatoes, for example). Cooking softens cellulose, making foods easier to chew and this, in turn, makes nutrients more available. However, **juicing** as we discussed above, also breaks down cellulose and frees the nutrients while retaining the **enzymes** that would be destroyed by cooking.

Unsprouted seeds contain enzyme inhibitors, which can be neutralized by cooking. However, soaking or sprouting the seeds also removes the enzyme inhibitors and **sprouts have a high concentration of vegetable enzymes and other nutrients**. Therefore, it is a good idea to soak your grains and beans in water for a minimum of 12 hours before eating them. Soaked grains and beans are called "pre-sprouts" and are much more digestible because the enzyme inhibitors have been deactivated. Allowing the seeds to sprout for three days allows the synthesis of new proteins, plus there is a dramatic increase in the vitamins and essential fatty acids within the sprouts.

Cooking food thoroughly kills bacteria and viruses, which is why with raw foods cleanliness becomes very important. The temperature of food and beverages also makes a difference to digestion. Warm food relaxes the stomach and aids digestion. **Cold food** and **beverages** contract the muscles of the stomach, **hindering proper digestion**.

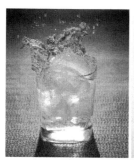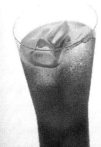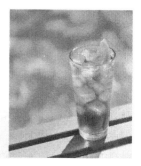

Actually it's quite dangerous for our digestive system to have cold drinks with meals. **Drink water or organic fruits and vegetable juices between meals and stop 15 min before the meal and start drinking again 40-45 min after the meal.** Beverages interfere with digestion because the **digestive liquid** and **enzymes** get carried **out** with the beverage rather than staying in the stomach. Also, drinking beverages might wash down food that has **not been properly broken** down through chewing and mixing with saliva in the mouth. This is certainly a way to create an environment to encourage colon cancer.

Lightly steaming vegetables warms and softens them while retaining most of their enzymes and nutrients.

Chapter 5

Cancer Cells DON'T breathe Oxygen

*"One must maintain **a little bit of summer**, even in the middle of winter."*

Henry David Thoreau

Dr Otto Warburg received the Nobel Prize in 1931 for the discovery that, unlike all other cells in the human body, cancer cells are effectively asphyxiated by oxygen within the body's tissues. **Cancer cells** are **anaerobic**, which means that they derive their energy without needing oxygen. It has been found that **Cancer cells cannot survive in the presence of high levels of oxygen** and this has given rise to a variety of successful cancer fighting treatments based on oxygenating the tissues, such as intravenous hydrogen peroxide, hyperbaric oxygen tank, and blood ozonation (Diamond, pages 912-927). Doing light exercises such as walking, treadmill, stationary bicycle or whatever possible at the moment with a deep breathing technique will provide more oxygen to the muscles therefore help the body to fight cancer.

As a preventive and self-treatment, breathing exercises (such as pranayama) and an abundance of fresh air provide a starting point. Most people do not breathe deeply, so they lose the benefit of much of their lung capacity. Most indoor air is ten times more polluted than outdoor air, yet we spend up to 90% of our time indoors. Indoor air in every room needs to be constantly refreshed from the outside. Do I need to mention the importance of not smoking? Aerobic exercise is useful both to oxygenate the tissues and to move the **lymph fluid around**.

Lymph is a colourless fluid that **bathes every cell in the body**. The body has two circulatory systems, one for **blood** and the other for **lymph**. **The heart circulates blood**, whereas **the lymph is circulated by physical exercise**. Many tissues depend on the lymph to provide nutrients (including oxygen) and carry off wastes. If the lymph does not circulate properly then the tissues suffocate while stewing in their own **acidic waste products (uric acid, lactic acid, etc.)**.

Chapter 6

Free Radicals and Acidity

*"You need to learn how to **select your thoughts** just the same way you select your clothes every day. This is a **power you can cultivate**. If you want to control things in your life so bad, work on the **mind**."*

Elizabeth Gilbert

So much has been written about free radicals and cancer. A harmful free radical is an **ion** that has a positive electrical charge. An electron has a negative electrical charge. Due to its positive charge, the free radical attracts electrons from other molecules, thereby damaging them. **Sources of free radicals include farm chemicals (fertilizers and pesticides), many prescription drugs, processed foods, cigarette smoke, environmental pollution, alcohol, electromagnetic radiation, and stress** (Sharma, pages 26-27).

In 1973, a study conducted by the Department of Occupational Health at Hebrew University-Hadassah

*Medical School in Jerusalem found that when cancerous breast tissue is compared with non-cancerous tissue from elsewhere in the same woman's body, the concentration of toxic chemicals such as DDT and PCBs was "**much increased in the malignant tissue compared to the normal breast and adjacent adipose tissue**."*

Areas in the body where flow of **lymph** is chronically impaired will experience an accumulation of cellular waste products and other toxic material. This leads to chronic **inflammation**, which in turn results in cancer. It is estimated that the average adult carries about 15 pounds of dried fecal matter in the colon.

Comparison of cancer tissue with healthy tissue from the same person shows that the **cancer tissue** has a much higher concentration of **toxic chemicals, pesticides, etc**. These substances not only build up in the body, but certain areas of the body seem to serve as a dumping ground.

Free radicals can damage any part of the cell, including the DNA. Free radical damage to the DNA is thought to be one of the causes of cancer. **In the absence of oxygen, the DNA self-repair mechanism does not function** (Diamond, page 1038), so it is no surprise that the DNA of cancerous tissue shows extensive free radical damage.

Antioxidants include selenium, glutathione, resveratrol, vitamins A, C and E, bioflavonoids, carotenoids, and

99

coenzyme Q10. Selenium is found in Brazil nuts and oatmeal. Many foods, particularly those of the cabbage family, are found to increase **glutathione** levels in the body. Selenium and glutathione work together to protect fatty tissues such as breast, liver and prostate. Glutathione protects and regulates the p53 tumour suppression gene that could potentially prevent half of all cancers. Vitamin C maintains the effectiveness of vitamin E as an antioxidant. Bioflavonoids are provided by green/blue/purple coloured foods (fruits, vegetables, berries, beans, spices, etc.). Carotenoids come from yellow/orange/red coloured foods. Many individual bioflavonoids and carotenoids have been shown to inhibit cancer growth, and when you eat a variety of foods containing bioflavonoids and carotenoids, they work together to produce a very powerful effect on cancer.

Other antioxidants and antioxidant sources include resveratrol (found in grape skins), propolis, zinc, green tea, turmeric, L-carnosine, and organic germanium. Prunes contain a very high concentration of antioxidants.

Oxidized (rancid) vegetable oils (corn oil, soy oil, soybean oil canola oil etc.), which break down under heat, look the same as non-oxidized vegetable oils, but the **oxidized oils produce masses of free radicals in your body**.

This is one of the reasons why I recommend you replace all vegetable cooking oils with **extra virgin olive oil or failing that, coconut oil**.

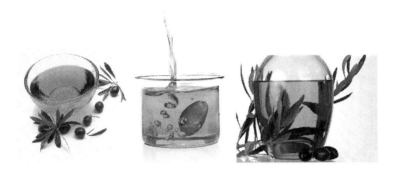

Other vegetable oils like Canola, Soybean Oil, etc., when heated over **60 C,** produce **masses of free radicals** so these should be avoided completely. For good health, be sure to eat at least 3 or 4 tablespoons of coconut oil every day if possible. Start with teaspoon amounts and work up. **Coconut oil** is very easy to digest and provides an ideal source of energy for sick people and healthy people.

For general DNA repair in your body, it is also useful for your diet to include foods containing abundant nucleotides that are the building blocks from which your body builds DNA and RNA.

Foods providing nucleotides:
Sardines
Brewer's yeast
Anchovies
Mackerel
Lentils
Most beans
Chlorella algae

Spirulina algae.

Please note that in addition to providing your body with a steady supply of nucleotides, removing excess **acidity** from the system and maintaining lower alkalinity will allow your body tissues to become aerobic and be responsive to the **DNA self-repair mechanism that can only function when alkalinity levels are normal.**

Essential Amino Acids

Amino acids are described as the "building blocks of protein," and they are important to the synthesis of proteins and the **overall functioning of the body**. In particular, there are 10 amino acids classified as **"essential,"** which means they are not naturally made by the human body. These amino acids must be acquired through the foods you eat, reports the University of Arizona Department of Biochemistry, or your body will begin to break down existing protein, such as **muscle tissue**. Unlike fat, amino acids can't be stored in the body for later use. Therefore, it is doubly important that you include these amino acids in your diet on a consistent basis.

Nuts

Nuts and **legumes** are abundant sources of amino acids. Walnuts, almonds, Brazil nuts, cashews and peanuts are all rich sources of the essential amino acid L-arginine. Arginine is known to **boost immune function**, assist in

muscle metabolism and muscle mass and enhance collagen production and bone growth. Almonds and cashews are also top sources of isoleucine, another essential amino acid that stabilizes blood sugar and increases energy. Almonds and peanuts also boast high levels of the amino acid phenylalanine, which is thought to enhance mood.

Wild Fish

Wild fish of any kind is another top source of many of the amino acids. Fatty fish such as salmon, tuna, herring and sardines are also rich in omega-3 fatty acids, which may have benefits in protecting against heart disease. Fish are abundant in the essential amino acids isoleucine, lysine and methionine.

Free-range eggs

Free-range eggs contain plentiful amounts of amino acids and are an excellent source of protein for relatively few calories. Eggs are good sources of the essential amino acids methionine, isoleucine and lysine. They are a good source of tryptophan, an essential amino acid involved in the production of the mood-enhancing neurotransmitter serotonin.

Whole eggs provide your body with a source of fat-soluble vitamins, including A, D and E, significant quantities of certain B complex vitamins, including B-6, B-12, folate and riboflavin and alkaline minerals such as **calcium, magnesium**, iron, zinc and **selenium**. As well as everything else you should eat them in moderation.

Let's have a look at the chart presenting the amount of mineral and vitamins as well as complete protein in nuts, seeds and whole grains for you to choose for the best muscle building blocks.

Best Alkalizing Nuts, Seeds and Grains chart with Mineral and Vitamin content

Nut/Seed	Protein/Fiber	Minerals	Vitamins
Almonds	1 ounce (23 whole nuts) of raw almonds contains 6.02 grams protein, 163 calories and 3.5 grams of dietary fiber.	Potassium - 200 mg Phosphorus - 137 mg Calcium - 75 mg Magnesium - 76 mg Iron - 1.05 mg Selenium - 0.7 mcg Zinc - 0.87 mg Manganese - 0.648 mg Copper - 0.282 mg Also contains a small amount of other minerals.	Vitamin B1 (thiamine) - 0.06 mg Vitamin B2 (riboflavin) - 0.287 mg Niacin - 0.96 mg Folate - 14 mcg Pantothenic Acid - 0.133 mg Vitamin B6 - 0.041 mg Vitamin E - 7.43 mg Contains some other vitamins in small amounts.
Amaranth	100 grams of cooked amaranth contain 3.8 grams protein, 102 calories and 2.1 grams dietary fiber.	Potassium - 135 mg Phosphorus - 148 mg Calcium - 47 mg Magnesium - 65 mg Iron - 2.1 mg Sodium - 6 mg Manganese - 0.854 mg Zinc - 0.86 mg Copper - 0.149 mg Selenium - 5.5 mcg Also contains trace amounts of other minerals.	Vitamin B1 (thiamine) - 0.015 mg Vitamin B2 (riboflavin) - 0.022 mg Niacin - 0.235 mg Vitamin B6 - 0.113 mg Folate - 22 mcg Vitamin E - 0.19 mg Contains some other vitamins in small amounts.
Barley (Pearled)	100 grams of cooked, pearled barley contain	Potassium - 93 mg Phosphorus - 54 mg Calcium - 11 mg	Vitamin B1 (thiamine) - 0.083 mg Vitamin B2 (riboflavin) -

	2.26 grams protein, 123 calories and 3.8 grams dietary fiber.	Magnesium - 22 mg Iron - 1.33 mg Sodium - 3 mg Manganese - 0.259 mg Zinc - 0.82 mg Copper - 0.105 mg Selenium - 8.6 mcg Also contains trace amounts of other minerals.	0.062 mg Niacin - 2.063 mg Pantothenic Acid - 0.135 mg Vitamin B6 - 0.115 mg Folate - 16 mcg Vitamin A - 7 IU Vitamin E - 0.01 mg Vitamin K - 0.8 mcg Contains some other vitamins in small amounts.
Brazil Nuts 	1 ounce (6 whole nuts) contains 4.06 grams of protein, 186 calories and 2.1 grams of fiber.	Potassium - 187 mg Phosphorus - 206 mg Calcium - 45 mg Magnesium - 107 mg Iron - 0.69 mg Sodium - 1 mg Manganese - 0.347 mg Zinc - 1.15 mg Copper - 0.494 mg Selenium - 543.5 mcg Also contains trace amounts of other minerals.	Vitamin C - 0.2 mg Vitamin B1 (thiamine) - 0.175 mg Vitamin B2 (riboflavin) - 0.01 mg Niacin - 0.084 mg Pantothenic Acid - 0.052 mg Vitamin B6 - 0.029 mg Folate - 6 mcg Vitamin E - 1.62 mg Contains some other vitamins in small amounts.
Buckwheat 	100 grams of buckwheat contain 13.25 grams protein, 343 calories and 10 grams dietary fiber.	Potassium - 460 mg Phosphorus - 347 mg Calcium - 18 mg Magnesium - 231 mg Iron - 2.2 mg Sodium - 1 mg Manganese - 1.3 mg Zinc - 2.4 mg Copper - 1.1 mg Selenium - 8.3 mcg Also contains trace amounts of other minerals.	Vitamin B1 (thiamine) - 0.101 mg Vitamin B2 (riboflavin) - 0.425 mg Niacin - 7.02 mg Pantothenic Acid - 1.233 mg Vitamin B6 - 0.21 mg Folate - 30 mcg Contains some other vitamins in small amounts.
Cashews 	One ounce of raw, unsalted cashew nuts contains 5.17 grams of protein, 157 calories and 0.94 grams of fiber.	Potassium - 187 mg Phosphorus - 168 mg Calcium - 10 mg Magnesium - 83 mg Iron - 1.89 mg Sodium - 3 mg Manganese - 0.469 mg Zinc - 1.64 mg Copper - 0.622 mg Selenium - 5.6 mcg Also contains trace amounts of other minerals.	Vitamin C - 0.1 mg Vitamin B1 (thiamine) - 0.12 mg Vitamin B2 (riboflavin) - 0.016 mg Niacin - 0.301 mg Pantothenic Acid - 0.245 mg Vitamin B6 - 0.118 mg Folate - 7 mcg Vitamin E - 0.26 mg Vitamin K - 9.7 mcg Contains some other vitamins in small amounts.

Chestnuts	Ten (10) roasted kernels with no salt added contain 2.66 grams protein, 206 calories and 4.3 grams fiber. (Note: chestnuts must be boiled or roasted before eating due to the high levels of tannic acid.)	Potassium - 497 mg Phosphorus - 90 mg Calcium - 24 mg Magnesium - 28 mg Iron - 0.76 mg Sodium - 2 mg Manganese - 0.991 mg Zinc - 0.48 mg Copper - 0.426 mg Selenium - 1 mcg Also contains trace amounts of other minerals.	Vitamin C - 21.8 mg Vitamin B1 (thiamine) - 0.204 mg Vitamin B2 (riboflavin) - 0.147 mg Niacin - 1.127 mg Pantothenic Acid - 0.465 mg Vitamin B6 - 0.417 mg Folate - 59 mcg Vitamin A - 20 IU Vitamin E - 0.42 mg Vitamin K - 6.6 mcg Contains some other vitamins in small amounts.
Coconut	One cup of raw, shredded coconut contains 2.66 grams of protein, 283 calories and 7.2 grams of dietary fiber.	Potassium - 285 mg Phosphorus - 90 mg Calcium - 11 mg Magnesium - 26 mg Iron - 1.94 mg Sodium - 16 mg Manganese - 1.2 mg Zinc - 0.88 mg Copper - 0.348 mg Selenium - 8.1 mcg Also contains trace amounts of other minerals.	Vitamin C - 2.6 mg Vitamin B1 (thiamine) - 0.053 mg Vitamin B2 (riboflavin) - 0.016 mg Niacin - 0.432 mg Pantothenic Acid - 0.24 mg Vitamin B6 - 0.043 mg Folate - 21 mcg Vitamin E - 0.19 mg Vitamin K - 0.2 mcg Contains some other vitamins in small amounts.
Flax Seed	One tablespoon of raw flax seeds contains 1.88 grams of protein, 55 calories and 2.8 grams of dietary fiber.	Potassium - 84 mg Phosphorus - 66 mg Calcium - 26 mg Magnesium - 40 mg Iron - 0.59 mg Sodium - 3 mg Manganese - 0.256 mg Zinc - 0.45 mg Copper - 0.126 mg Selenium - 2.6 mcg Also contains trace amounts of other minerals.	Vitamin C 0.1 mg Vitamin B1 (thiamine) - 0.169 mg Vitamin B2 (riboflavin) - 0.017 mg Niacin - 0.317 mg Pantothenic Acid - 0.101 mg Vitamin B6 - 0.049 mg Folate - 9 mcg Vitamin E - 0.03 mg Vitamin K - 0.4 mcg Contains some other vitamins in small amounts.
Hazelnuts	One ounce (21 whole kernels) of hazelnuts contains 4.24 grams of protein, 178 calories and 2.7	Potassium - 193 mg Phosphorus - 82 mg Calcium - 32 mg Magnesium - 46 mg Iron - 1.33 mg Manganese - 1.751 mg Zinc - 0.69 mg	Vitamin C - 1.8 mg Vitamin B1 (thiamine) - 0.182 mg Vitamin B2 (riboflavin) - 0.032 mg Niacin - 0.51 mg Pantothenic Acid - 0.26

	grams of dietary fiber.	Copper - 0.489 mg Selenium - 0.7 mcg Also contains trace amounts of other minerals.	mg Vitamin B6 - 0.16 mg Folate - 32 mcg Vitamin A - 6 IU Vitamin E - 4.26 mg Vitamin K - 4 mcg Contains some other vitamins in small amounts.
Macadamias	One once (10-12 kernels) of raw macadamia nuts contains 2.24 grams protein, 204 calories and 2.4 grams fiber.	Potassium - 104 mg Phosphorus - 53 mg Calcium - 24 mg Magnesium - 37 mg Iron - 1.05 mg Sodium - 1 mg Manganese - 1.171 mg Zinc - 0.37 mg Copper - 0.214 mg Selenium - 1 mcg Also contains trace amounts of other minerals.	Vitamin C - 0.3 mg Vitamin B1 (thiamine) - 0.339 mg Vitamin B2 (riboflavin) - 0.046 mg Niacin - 0.701 mg Pantothenic Acid - 0.215 mg Vitamin B6 - 0.078 mg Folate - 3 mcg Vitamin E - 0.15 mg Contains some other vitamins in small amounts.
Millet	100 grams of cooked millet contain 3.51 grams protein, 119 calories and 1.3 grams dietary fiber.	Potassium - 62 mg Phosphorus - 100 mg Calcium - 3 mg Magnesium - 44 mg Iron - 0.63 mg Sodium - 2 mg Manganese - 0.272 mg Zinc - 0.91 mg Copper - 0.161 mg Selenium - 0.9 mcg Also contains trace amounts of other minerals.	Vitamin B1 (thiamine) - 0.106 mg Vitamin B2 (riboflavin) - 0.082 mg Niacin - 1.33 mg Pantothenic Acid - 0.171 mg Vitamin B6 - 0.108 mg Folate - 19 mcg Vitamin A - 3 IU Vitamin E - 0.02 mg Vitamin K - 0.3 mcg Contains some other vitamins in small amounts.
Oats	100 grams of oats contain grams 16.89 protein, 389 calories and 10.6 grams dietary fiber.	Potassium - 429 mg Phosphorus - 523 mg Calcium - 54 mg Magnesium - 177 mg Iron - 4.72 mg Sodium - 2 mg Manganese - 4.916 mg Zinc - 3.97 mg Copper - 0.626 mg Also contains trace amounts of other minerals.	Vitamin B1 (thiamine) - 0.763 mg Vitamin B2 (riboflavin) - 0.139 mg Niacin - 0.961 mg Pantothenic Acid - 1.349 mg Vitamin B6 - 0.119 mg Folate - 56 mcg Contains some other vitamins in small amounts.
peanuts	One ounce of dry roasted peanuts contains	Potassium -187 mg Phosphorus - 101 mg Calcium - 15 mg	Vitamin B1 (thiamine) - 0.124 mg Vitamin B2 (riboflavin) -

	6.71 grams of protein, 166 calories and 2.3 grams of dietary fiber.	Magnesium - 50 mg Iron - 0.64 mg Sodium - 2 mg Manganese - 0.591 mg Zinc - 0.94 mg Copper - 0.190 mg Selenium - 2.1 mcg Also contains trace amounts of other minerals.	0.028 mg Niacin - 3.834 mg Pantothenic Acid - 0.395 mg Vitamin B6 - 0.073 mg Folate - 41 mcg Vitamin E - 1.96 mg Contains some other vitamins in small amounts.
Pecans	One ounce (19 halves) of raw pecans contains 2.6 grams protein, 196 calories and 2.7 grams fiber.	Potassium - 116 mg Phosphorus - 79 mg Calcium - 20 mg Magnesium - 34 mg Iron - 0.72 mg Manganese - 1.276 mg Zinc - 1.28 mg Copper - 0.34 mg Selenium - 1.1 mcg Also contains trace amounts of other minerals.	Vitamin C - 0.3 mg Vitamin B1 (thiamine) - 0.187 mg Vitamin B2 (riboflavin) - 0.01 mg Niacin - 0.331 mg Pantothenic Acid - 0.245 mg Vitamin B6 - 0.06 mg Folate - 6 mcg Vitamin A - 16 IU Vitamin E - 0.4 mg Vitamin K - 1 mcg Contains some other vitamins in small amounts.
Pine Nuts / Pignolias	One ounce of pine nuts (167 kernels) contains 3.88 grams of protein, 191 calories and 1.0 grams of dietary fiber.	Potassium - 169 mg Phosphorus - 163 mg Calcium - 5 mg Magnesium - 71 mg Iron - 1.57 mg Sodium - 1 mg Manganese - 2.495 mg Zinc - 1.83 mg Copper - 0.375 mg Selenium - 0.2 mcg Also contains trace amounts of other minerals.	Vitamin C - 0.2 mg Vitamin B1 (thiamine) - 0.103 mg Vitamin B2 (riboflavin) - 0.064 mg Niacin - 1.244 mg Pantothenic Acid - 0.089 mg Vitamin B6 - 0.027 mg Folate - 10 mcg Vitamin A - 8 IU Vitamin E - 2.65 mg Vitamin K - 15.3 mcg Contains some other vitamins in small amounts.
Pistachios	One ounce of dry roasted pistachio nuts (no salt) (49 kernels) contains 6.05 grams of protein, 162 calories and 2.9 grams of dietary fiber.	Potassium - 295 mg Phosphorus - 137 mg Calcium - 31 mg Magnesium - 34 mg Iron - 1.19 mg Sodium - 3 mg Manganese - 0.361 mg Zinc - 0.65 mg Copper - 0.376 mg Selenium - 2.6 mcg Also contains trace amounts of	Vitamin C - 0.7 mg Vitamin B1 (thiamine) - 0.238 mg Vitamin B2 (riboflavin) - 0.045 mg Niacin - 0.404 mg Pantothenic Acid - 0.145 mg Vitamin B6 - 0.361 mg Folate - 14 mcg Vitamin A - 74 IU Vitamin E - 0.55 mg

		other minerals.	Vitamin K - 3.7 mcg Contains some other vitamins in small amounts.
Pumpkin Seeds	One ounce of roasted pumpkin or squash seed kernels (no salt) contains 8.46 grams of protein, 163 calories and 1.8 grams of dietary fiber.	Potassium - 223 mg Phosphorus - 333 mg Calcium - 15 mg Magnesium - 156 mg Iron - 2.29 mg Sodium - 5 mg Manganese - 1.273 mg Zinc - 2.17 mg Copper - 0.361 mg Selenium - 2.7 mcg Also contains trace amounts of other minerals.	Vitamin C - 0.5 mg Vitamin B1 (thiamine) - 0.02 mg Vitamin B2 (riboflavin) - 0.043 mg Niacin - 1.256 mg Pantothenic Acid - 0.162 mg Vitamin B6 - 0.028 mg Folate - 16 mcg Vitamin A - 2 IU Vitamin E - 0.16 mg Vitamin K - 1.3 mcg Contains some other vitamins in small amounts.
Quinoa	100 grams of cooked quinoa contain 4.4 grams protein, 120 calories and 2.8 grams dietary fiber.	Potassium - 172 mg Phosphorus - 152 mg Calcium - 17 mg Magnesium - 64 mg Iron - 1.49 mg Sodium - 7 mg Manganese - 0.631 mg Zinc - 1.09 mg Copper - 0.192 mg Selenium - 2.8 mcg Also contains trace amounts of other minerals.	Vitamin B1 (thiamine) - 0.107 mg Vitamin B2 (riboflavin) - 0.11 mg Niacin - 0.412 mg Vitamin B6 - 0.123 mg Folate - 42 mcg Vitamin A - 5 IU Vitamin E - 0.63 mg Contains some other vitamins in small amounts.
Rice - Brown	100 grams of cooked brown rice contain 2.32 grams of protein, 112 calories and 1.8 grams of dietary fiber.	Potassium - 79 mg Phosphorus - 77 mg Calcium - 10 mg Magnesium - 44 mg Iron - 0.53 mg Sodium - 1 mg Manganese - 1.097 mg Zinc - 0.62 mg Copper - 0.081 mg Also contains trace amounts of other minerals.	Vitamin B1 (thiamine) - 0.102 mg Vitamin B2 (riboflavin) - 0.012 mg Niacin - 1.33 mg Pantothenic Acid - 0.392 mg Vitamin B6 - 0.149 mg Folate - 4 mcg Contains some other vitamins in small amounts.
Rice - Wild	100 grams of cooked wild rice contain 3.99 grams of protein, 101 calories and 1.8 grams of dietary fiber	Potassium - 101 mg Phosphorus - 82 mg Calcium - 3 mg Magnesium - 32 mg Iron - 0.6 mg Sodium - 3 mg Manganese - 0.282 mg Zinc - 1.34 mg	Vitamin B1 (thiamine) - 0.052 mg Vitamin B2 (riboflavin) - 0.087 mg Niacin - 1.287 mg Pantothenic Acid - 0.154 mg Vitamin B6 - 0.135 mg

		Copper - 0.121 mg Selenium - 0.8 mcg Also contains trace amounts of other minerals.	Folate - 26 mcg Vitamin A - 3 IU Vitamin E - 0.24 mg Vitamin K - 0.5 mcg Contains some other vitamins in small amounts.
Rye	100 grams of rye contain 10.34 grams protein, 338 calories and 14.6 grams dietary fiber.	Potassium - 510 mg Phosphorus - 332 mg Calcium - 24 mg Magnesium - 110 mg Iron - 2.63 mg Sodium - 2 mg Manganese - 2.577 mg Zinc - 2.65 mg Copper - 0.367 mg Selenium - 13.9 mcg Also contains trace amounts of other minerals.	Vitamin B1 (thiamine) - 0.316 mg Vitamin B2 (riboflavin) - 0.251 mg Niacin - 4.27 mg Pantothenic Acid - 1.456 mg Vitamin B6 - 0.294 mg Folate - 38 mcg Vitamin A - 11 IU Vitamin E - 0.85 mg Vitamin K - 5.9 mcg Contains some other vitamins in small amounts.
Sesame Seeds	One tablespoon of dried sesame seeds (no salt) contains 1.6 grams of protein, 52 calories and 1.1 grams of dietary fiber.	Potassium - 42 mg Phosphorus - 57 mg Calcium - 88 mg Magnesium - 32 mg Iron - 1.31 mg Sodium - 1 mg Manganese - 0.221 mg Zinc - 0.7 mg Copper - 0.367 mg Selenium - 3.1 mcg Also contains trace amounts of other minerals.	Vitamin B1 (thiamine) - 0.071 mg Vitamin B2 (riboflavin) - 0.022 mg Niacin - 0.406 mg Pantothenic Acid - 0.005 mg Vitamin B6 - 0.071 mg Folate - 9 mcg Vitamin A - 1 IU Vitamin E - 0.02 mg Contains some other vitamins in small amounts.
Spelt	100 grams of cooked, spelt contain 5.5 grams protein, 127 calories and 3.9 grams dietary fiber.	Potassium - 143 mg Phosphorus - 150 mg Calcium - 10 mg Magnesium - 49 mg Iron - 1.67 mg Sodium - 5 mg Manganese - 1.091 mg Zinc - 1.25 mg Copper - 0.215 mg Selenium - 4 mcg Also contains trace amounts of other minerals.	Vitamin B1 (thiamine) - 0.103 mg Vitamin B2 (riboflavin) - 0.03 mg Niacin - 2.57 mg Vitamin B6 - 0.08 mg Folate - 13 mcg Vitamin A - 4 IU Vitamin E - 0.26 mg Contains some other vitamins in small amounts.
Sunflower Seeds	One ounce of sunflower seed kernels, dry-roasted without	Potassium - 241 mg Phosphorus - 327 mg Calcium - 20 mg Magnesium - 37 mg	Vitamin C - 0.4 mg Vitamin B1 (thiamine) - 0.03 mg Vitamin B2 (riboflavin) -

	salt contains 5.48 grams of protein, 165 calories and 3.1 grams of dietary fiber.	Iron - 1.08 mg Sodium - 1 mg Manganese - 0.598 mg Zinc - 1.5 mg Copper - 0.519 mg Selenium - 22.5 mcg Also contains trace amounts of other minerals.	0.07 mg Niacin - 1.996 mg Pantothenic Acid - 1.996 mg Vitamin B6 - 0.228 mg Folate - 67 mcg Vitamin A - 3 IU Vitamin E - 7.4 mg Vitamin K - 0.8 mcg Contains some other vitamins in small amounts.
Walnuts 	1 ounce (14 halves) English walnuts contain 4.32 mg protein, 185 calories and 1.9 mg fiber.	Potassium - 125 mg Phosphorus - 98 mg Calcium - 28 mg Magnesium - 45 mg Iron - 0.82 mg Sodium - 1 mg Manganese - 0.968 mg Zinc - 0.88 mg Copper - 0.45 mg Selenium - 1.4 mcg Also contains trace amounts of other minerals.	Vitamin C - 0.4 mg Vitamin B1 (thiamine) - 0.097 mg Vitamin B2 (riboflavin) - 0.043 mg Niacin - 0.319 mg Pantothenic Acid - 0.162 mg Vitamin B6 - 0.152 mg Folate - 28 mcg Vitamin A - 6 IU Vitamin E - 0.2 mg Vitamin K - 0.8 mcg Contains some other vitamins in small amounts.
Wheat - Durum 	100 grams of durum wheat contain 13.68 grams protein and 339 calories.	Potassium - 431 mg Phosphorus - 508 mg Calcium - 34 mg Magnesium - 144 mg Iron - 3.52 mg Sodium - 2 mg Manganese - 3.012 mg Zinc - 4.16 mg Copper - 0.553 mg Selenium - 89.4 mcg Also contains trace amounts of other minerals.	Vitamin B1 (thiamine) - 0.419 mg Vitamin B2 (riboflavin) - 0.121 mg Niacin - 6.738 mg Pantothenic Acid - 0.935 mg Vitamin B6 - 0.419 mg Folate - 43 mcg Contains some other vitamins in small amounts.
Wheat - Hard Red 	100 grams of hard red wheat contain 15.40 grams protein, 329 calories and 12.2 grams of dietary fiber.	Potassium - 340 mg Phosphorus - 332 mg Calcium - 25 mg Magnesium - 124 mg Iron - 3.6 mg Sodium - 2 mg Manganese - 4.055 mg Zinc - 2.78 mg Copper - 0.41 mg Selenium - 70.7 mcg Also contains trace amounts of other minerals.	Vitamin B1 (thiamine) - 0.504 mg Vitamin B2 (riboflavin) - 0.11 mg Niacin - 5.71 mg Pantothenic Acid - 0.935 mg Vitamin B6 - 0.336 mg Folate - 43 mcg Vitamin A - 9 IU Vitamin E - 1.01 mg Vitamin K - 1.9 mcg Contains some other

			vitamins in small amounts.
Wheat - Hard White(whole)	100 grams of hard white wheat contain 11.31 grams protein, 342 calories and 12.2 grams dietary fiber.	Potassium - 432 mg Phosphorus - 355 mg Calcium - 32 mg Magnesium - 93 mg Iron - 4.56 mg Sodium - 2 mg Manganese - 3.821 mg Zinc - 3.33 mg Copper - 0.363 mg Also contains trace amounts of other minerals.	Vitamin B1 (thiamine) - 0.387 mg Vitamin B2 (riboflavin) - 0.108 mg Niacin - 4.381 mg Pantothenic Acid - 0.954 mg Vitamin B6 - 0.368 mg Folate - 38 mcg Vitamin A - 9 IU Vitamin E - 1.01 mg Vitamin K - 1.9 mcg Contains some other vitamins in small amounts.

Chapter 7

What you should Know about Food Containing Soy – the full details

*"Anyone who stops learning is old, whether at twenty or eighty. Anyone who keeps learning stays young. **The greatest thing in life is to keep your mind young.**"*

Henry Ford

Soybeans contain natural toxins that inhibit protein digestion in the body and should be completely avoided in your foods going forward. Only a few decades ago, unfermented soybean foods were considered unfit to eat - even in Asia. These days, people all over the world have been fooled into thinking that unfermented soy foods like soymilk and soy protein are somehow "health foods". If they only knew the real truth!

The soybean did not serve as a food until the discovery of fermentation techniques, sometime during the Chou Dynasty. The first soy foods were fermented products like tempeh, natto, miso and soy sauce.

At a later date, possibly in the 2nd century BC, Chinese scientists discovered that a puree of cooked soybeans could be precipitated with calcium sulphate or magnesium sulphate (plaster of Paris or Epsom salts) to make a smooth, pale curd - tofu or bean curd. The use of fermented and precipitated soy products soon spread to other parts of the Orient, notably Japan and Indonesia.

Growth-depressant compounds are deactivated during the process of fermentation, so once the Chinese discovered how to ferment the soybean, they began to incorporate soy foods into their diets.

The Chinese NEVER ate large amounts of unfermented soy foods or soymilk.

The Chinese did not eat unfermented soybeans as they did other legumes such as lentils because the soybean contains large quantities of natural toxins or "anti nutrients". First among them are potent enzyme inhibitors that **block the action of trypsin and other enzymes vital for protein digestion.**

These inhibitors are large, tightly folded proteins that are not completely deactivated during ordinary cooking. They can produce serious gastric distress, reduced protein digestion and chronic deficiencies in amino acid uptake. In test animals, diets high in trypsin inhibitors cause enlargement and pathological conditions of the pancreas, including cancer.

Soybeans also contain haemagglutinin, a clot-promoting substance that causes red blood cells to clump together. Trypsin inhibitors and haemagglutinin are growth inhibitors. Weaned rats fed soy containing these antinutrients fail to grow normally.

Soy also contains **goitrogens** - substances that depress **thyroid function**.

Although soy has been known to suppress thyroid function for over 60 years, and although scientists have identified the goitrogenic component of soy as the so-called "beneficial isoflavones", the industry insists that soy depresses thyroid function only in the absence of iodine.

The University of Alabama at Birmingham reports a case in which consumption of a soy protein dietary supplement decreased the absorption of thyroxin. The patient had undergone thyroid surgery and needed to take thyroid hormone. Higher oral doses of thyroid hormone were needed when she consumed soy -- she presumably used iodized salt so iodine intake did not prevent the goitrogenic effects of soy.

A very large percentage of soy is genetically modified and it also has one of the highest percentages of **contamination by pesticides** of any of our foods.

Soybeans are high in phytic acid, present in the bran or hulls of all seeds. Phytic acid is a substance that can block the uptake of essential minerals - **calcium, magnesium, copper, iron and especially zinc - in the intestinal tract.** The soybean has one of the highest phytate levels of any grain or legume that has been studied, and the phytates in soy are highly resistant to normal phytate-reducing techniques such as long, slow cooking. Only a long period of fermentation will significantly reduce the phytate content of soybeans.

Soy Protein Isolate is an Industrially Produced Food -- Far from Natural or Healthy!

SPI is not something you can make in your own kitchen. Production takes place in industrial factories where slurry of soy beans is first mixed with an alkaline solution to remove fibre, then precipitated and separated using an acid wash and, finally, neutralized in an alkaline solution.

Acid washing in aluminium tanks leaches high levels of aluminium into the final product. The resultant curds are spray - dried at high temperatures to produce a high-protein powder. A final indignity to the original soybean is high-temperature; high-pressure extrusion processing of soy protein isolates to produce textured vegetable protein.

In feeding experiments, the use of SPI increased requirements for vitamins E, K, D and B12 and created deficiency symptoms of calcium, magnesium, manganese, molybdenum, copper, iron and zinc. Phytic acid remaining in these soy products greatly inhibits zinc and iron absorption; test animals fed SPI develop enlarged organs, particularly the **pancreas and thyroid gland**, and increased deposition of fatty acids in the liver.

Yet soy protein isolate and textured vegetable protein (TVP) are used extensively in school lunch programs, commercial baked goods, **diet beverages** and **fast food** products. They are heavily promoted in third world countries and form the basis of many food give-away programs.

Soy has the potential to disrupt the **digestive, immune and endocrine systems** of the human body and its role in rising rates of infertility, hypothyroidism and some types of **cancer including thyroid** and **pancreatic cancers**.

Soy is also highly **allergenic**. Most experts now place soy protein among the top eight allergens of all foods, and some rate it in the top six or even top four. Allergic reactions to soy are increasingly common, ranging from mild to life threatening, and some fatalities have been reported.

At the same time the variety of beans and peas widely available for us to enjoy the taste while nourishing the body is plenty to choose from:

Best Alkalizing Beans and Peas with Mineral and Vitamin content

Beans/Peas	Protein/Fiber	Minerals	Vitamins
Adzuki Beans	100 grams of Adzuki Beans, boiled without salt contain 7.52 grams protein, 128 calories and 7.3 grams dietary fiber.	Potassium - 532 mg Phosphorus - 168 mg Calcium - 28 mg Magnesium - 52 mg Iron - 2 mg Sodium - 8 mg Selenium - 1.2 mcg Zinc - 1.77 mg Manganese - 0.573 mg Copper - 0.298 mg Also contains a small amount of other minerals.	Vitamin B1 (thiamine) - 0.115 mg Vitamin B2 (riboflavin) - 0.064 mg Niacin - 0.717 mg Folate - 121 mcg Pantothenic Acid - 0.430 mg Vitamin B6 - 0.096 mg Vitamin A - 6 IU Contains some other vitamins in small amounts.
Black Beans	100 grams of Black Beans, boiled without salt, contain 8.86 grams protein, 132 calories and 8.7 grams of dietary fiber.	Potassium - 355 mg Phosphorus - 140 mg Calcium - 27 mg Magnesium - 70 mg Iron - 2.1 mg Sodium - 1 mg Manganese - 0.444 mg Zinc - 1.12 mg Copper - 0.209 mg Selenium - 1.2 mcg Also contains trace amounts of other minerals.	Vitamin B1 (thiamine) - 0.244 mg Vitamin B2 (riboflavin) - 0.059 mg Niacin - 0.505 mg Pantothenic Acid - 0.242 mg Vitamin B6 - 0.069 mg Folate - 149 mcg Vitamin A - 6 IU Contains some other vitamins in small amounts.
Black Eye or Cow Peas	100 grams of cooked, Black Eye Peas contain 7.73 grams protein, 116 calories and 6.5 grams dietary fiber.	Potassium - 278 mg Phosphorus - 156 mg Calcium - 24 mg Magnesium - 53 mg Iron - 2.51 mg Sodium - 4 mg Manganese - 0.475 mg Zinc - 1.29 mg Copper - 0.268 mg	Vitamin B1 (thiamine) - 0.202 mg Vitamin B2 (riboflavin) - 0.055 mg Niacin - 0.495 mg Pantothenic Acid - 0.411 mg Vitamin B6 - 0.1 mg Folate - 208 mcg

		Selenium - 2.5 mcg Also contains trace amounts of other minerals.	Vitamin A - 15 IU Vitamin E - 0.28 mg Vitamin K - 1.7 mcg Contains some other vitamins in small amounts.
Broad or Fava Beans	100 grams of Broad Beans contain 7.6 grams of protein, 110 calories and 5.4 grams of dietary fiber.	Potassium - 268 mg Phosphorus - 125 mg Calcium - 36 mg Magnesium - 43 mg Iron - 1.5 mg Sodium - 5 mg Manganese - 0.421 mg Zinc - 1.01 mg Copper - 0.259 mg Selenium - 2.6 mcg Also contains trace amounts of other minerals.	Vitamin C - 0.3 mg Vitamin B1 (thiamine) - 0.097 mg Vitamin B2 (riboflavin) - 0.089 mg Niacin - 0.711 mg Pantothenic Acid - 0.157 mg Vitamin B6 - 0.072 mg Folate - 104 mcg Vitamin A - 15 IU Vitamin E - 0.02 mg Vitamin K - 2.9 mcg Contains some other vitamins in small amounts.
Edamame	100 grams of frozen, unprepared Edamame contain 10.25 grams protein, 110 calories and 4.8 grams dietary fiber.	Potassium - 482 mg Phosphorus - 161 mg Calcium - 60 mg Magnesium - 61 mg Iron - 2.11 mg Sodium - 6 mg Manganese - 1.01 mg Zinc - 1.32 mg Copper - 0.324 mg Also contains trace amounts of other minerals.	Vitamin C - 9.7 mg Vitamin B1 (thiamine) - 0.15 mg Vitamin B2 (riboflavin) - 0.265 mg Niacin - 0.925 mg Pantothenic Acid - 0.535 mg Vitamin B6 - 0.135 mg Folate - 303 mcg Vitamin E - 0.72 mg Vitamin K - 31.4 mcg Contains some other vitamins in small amounts.
Chick Peas/Garbanzo Beans	100 grams of Garbanzo Beans, boiled without salt contain 8.86 grams protein, 164 calories and 7.6 grams of fiber.	Potassium - 291 mg Phosphorus - 168 mg Calcium - 49 mg Magnesium - 48 mg Iron - 2.89 mg Sodium - 7 mg Manganese - 1.03 mg Zinc - 1.53 mg Copper - 0.352 mg Selenium - 3.7 mcg Also contains trace amounts of other minerals.	Vitamin C - 1.3 mg Vitamin B1 (thiamine) - 0.116 mg Vitamin B2 (riboflavin) - 0.063 mg Niacin - 0.526 mg Pantothenic Acid - 0.286 mg Vitamin B6 - 0.139 mg Folate - 172 mcg Vitamin A - 27 IU Vitamin E - 0.35 mg Vitamin K - 4 mcg Contains some other

			vitamins in small amounts.
Kidney or Red Beans	100 grams of Kidney Beans, boiled without salt, contain 8.67 grams of protein, 127 calories and 7.3 grams dietary fiber.	Potassium - 403 mg Phosphorus - 142 mg Calcium - 28 mg Magnesium - 45 mg Iron - 2.94 mg Sodium - 2 mg Manganese - 0.477 mg Zinc - 1.07 mg Copper - 0.242 mg Selenium - 1.2 mcg Also contains trace amounts of other minerals.	Vitamin C - 1.2 mg Vitamin B1 (thiamine) - 0.216 mg Vitamin B2 (riboflavin) - 0.058 mg Niacin - 0.578 mg Pantothenic Acid - 0.22 mg Vitamin B6 - 0.12 mg Folate - 130 mcg Vitamin E - 0.03 mg Vitamin K - 8.4 mcg Contains some other vitamins in small amounts.
Lima Beans	100 grams of Lima Beans, boiled without salt contain 7.80 grams of protein, 115 calories and 7.0 grams of dietary fiber.	Potassium - 508 mg Phosphorus - 111 mg Calcium - 17 mg Magnesium - 43 mg Iron - 2.39 mg Sodium - 2 mg Manganese - 0.516 mg Zinc - 0.95 mg Copper - 0.235 mg Selenium - 4.5 mcg Also contains trace amounts of other minerals.	Vitamin B1 (thiamine) - 0.161 mg Vitamin B2 (riboflavin) - 0.055 mg Niacin - 0.421 mg Pantothenic Acid - 0.422 mg Vitamin B6 - 0.161 mg Folate - 83 mcg Vitamin E - 0.18 mg Vitamin K - 2 mcg Contains some other vitamins in small amounts.
Mung Beans	100 grams of Mung Beans, boiled without salt, have 7.02 grams of protein, 105 calories and 7.6 grams of dietary fiber.	Potassium - 266 mg Phosphorus - 99 mg Calcium - 27 mg Magnesium - 48 mg Iron - 1.4 mg Sodium - 2 mg Manganese - 0.298 mg Zinc - 0.84 mg Copper - 0.156 mg Selenium - 2.5 mcg Also contains trace amounts of other minerals.	Vitamin B1 (thiamine) - 0.164 mg Vitamin B2 (riboflavin) - 0.061 mg Niacin - 0.577 mg Pantothenic Acid - 0.41 mg Vitamin B6 - 0.067 mg Folate - 159 mcg Vitamin A - 24 IU Vitamin E - 0.15 mg Vitamin K - 2.7 mcg Contains some other vitamins in small amounts.

Navy Beans	100 grams Navy Beans, boiled without salt contain 8.23 grams proteins, 140 calories and 10.5 grams of dietary fiber.	Potassium - 389 mg Phosphorus - 144 mg Calcium - 69 mg Magnesium - 53 mg Iron - 2.36 mg Manganese - 0.527 mg Zinc - 1.03 mg Copper - 0.21 mg Selenium - 2.9 mcg Also contains trace amounts of other minerals.	Vitamin C - 0.9 mg Vitamin B1 (thiamine) - 0.237 mg Vitamin B2 (riboflavin) - 0.066 mg Niacin - 0.649 mg Pantothenic Acid - 0.266 mg Vitamin B6 - 0.138 mg Folate - 140 mcg Vitamin E - 0.01 mg Vitamin K - 0.6 mcg Contains some other vitamins in small amounts.
Pigeon Peas	100 grams of Pigeon Peas boiled without salt contain 6.76 grams proteins, 121 calories and 6.7 grams of dietary fiber.	Potassium -384 mg Phosphorus - 119 mg Calcium - 43 mg Magnesium - 46 mg Iron - 1.11 mg Sodium - 5 mg Manganese - 0.501 mg Zinc - 0.9 mg Copper - 0.269 mg Selenium - 2.9 mcg Also contains trace amounts of other minerals.	Vitamin B1 (thiamine) - 0.146 mg Vitamin B2 (riboflavin) - 0.059 mg Niacin - 0.781 mg Pantothenic Acid - 0.319 mg Vitamin B6 - 0.05 mg Folate - 111 mcg Vitamin A - 3 IU Contains some other vitamins in small amounts.
Pinto Beans	100 grams of Pinto Beans, boiled without salt, contain 9.01 grams of protein, 143 calories and 9 grams fiber.	Potassium - 436 mg Phosphorus - 147 mg Calcium - 46 mg Magnesium - 50 mg Iron - 2.09 mg Sodium - 1 mg Manganese - 0.453 mg Zinc - 0.98 mg Copper - 0.219 mg Selenium - 6.2 mcg Also contains trace amounts of other minerals.	Vitamin C - 0.8 mg Vitamin B1 (thiamine) - 0.193 mg Vitamin B2 (riboflavin) - 0.062 mg Niacin - 0.318 mg Pantothenic Acid - 0.21 mg Vitamin B6 - 0.229 mg Folate - 172 mcg Vitamin E - 0.94 mg Vitamin K - 3.5 mcg Contains some other vitamins in small amounts.

Split Peas	100 grams of Split Peas, boiled, without salt contain 8.34 grams protein, 118 calories and 8.3 grams dietary fiber.	Potassium - 362 mg Phosphorus - 99 mg Calcium - 14 mg Magnesium - 36 mg Iron - 1.29 mg Sodium - 2 mg Manganese - 0.396 mg Zinc - 1 mg Copper - 0.181 mg Selenium - 0.6 mcg Also contains trace amounts of other minerals.	Vitamin C - 0.4 mg Vitamin B1 (thiamine) - 0.19 mg Vitamin B2 (riboflavin) - 0.056 mg Niacin - 0.89 mg Pantothenic Acid - 0.595 mg Vitamin B6 - 0.048 mg Folate - 65 mcg Vitamin A - 7 IU Vitamin E - 0.03 mg Vitamin K - 5 mcg Contains some other vitamins in small amounts.
White Beans	100 grams White Beans, boiled without salt, contain 8.97 grams protein, 142 calories and 10.4 grams dietary fiber.	Potassium - 463 mg Phosphorus - 169 mg Calcium - 73 mg Magnesium - 68 mg Iron - 2.84 mg Manganese - 0.51 mg Zinc - 1.09 mg Copper - 0.149 mg Selenium - 1.3 mcg Also contains trace amounts of other minerals.	Vitamin B1 (thiamine) - 0.236 mg Vitamin B2 (riboflavin) - 0.059 mg Niacin - 0.272 mg Pantothenic Acid - 0.251 mg Vitamin B6 - 0.127 mg Folate - 137 mcg Contains some other vitamins in small amounts.
Winged Beans	100 grams Winged Beans, boiled without salt, contain 10.62 grams of protein and 147 calories.	Potassium - 280 mg Phosphorus - 153 mg Calcium - 142 mg Magnesium - 54 mg Iron - 4.33 mg Sodium - 13 mg Manganese - 1.199 mg Zinc - 1.44 mg Copper - 0.773 mg Selenium - 2.9 mcg Also contains trace amounts of other minerals.	Vitamin B1 (thiamine) - 0.295 mg Vitamin B2 (riboflavin) - 0.129 mg Niacin - 0.83 mg Pantothenic Acid - 0.156 mg Vitamin B6 - 0.047 mg Folate - 10 mcg Contains some other vitamins in small amounts.

Chapter 8

What Keeps the Hunza People FREE of Cancer

*There are two ways to live **your life**. One is as though nothing is a miracle. The other is as **though everything is a miracle** –*

Albert Einstein.

How would you like to live in a land where cancer does not exist? A land where an optometrist discovers to his amazement that everyone has perfect 20-20 vision? A land where cardiologists cannot find a single trace of **coronary heart disease**? How would you like to live in a land where no one ever gets **heart ailments, cancer, arthritis, high blood pressure, diabetes, tuberculosis, hay fever, asthma, liver trouble, gall bladder trouble, constipation, ulcers, appendicitis, and gout**? A land where men of 80 and 90 father children, and there's nothing unusual about men and women enjoying vigorous life at the age of 100 or 120?

Where does such an apparently magical place like that exist on our beautiful planet Earth?

A tiny little hidden region in the mountains, a place called Hunza in the high passes between the borders of China, Russia, India and Pakistan. Now ask yourself a few questions:

1. Are you willing to live 20,000 feet up in the mountains, almost completely out of touch with the rest of the world?

2. Are you ready to go outside in every kind of weather to tend your small mountainside garden, while keeping your ears open for an impending avalanche?

3. Are you prepared to give up not only every luxury of civilization, but even reading, writing and Internet access?

Quite major change requirements, right? At the same time if you want the benefits of the pure air that whips by the icy cathedrals of the Himalayan Mountains, the pure water that dances down from glaciers formed at 25,000 feet, and the mental and spiritual peace that comes from living in a land where there is no crime, taxes, social striving or generation gaps, no banks or stores-in fact-no money- where are you going to find it outside of Hunza?

But don't give up! Not yet, because there is still one more question to be answered. Which is: **are you prepared to eat the kind of food the Hunza people eat**? If you are, then you can rightfully expect to give yourself at least some measure of the **super health** and **resistance** to degenerative

124

disease, which the Hunzakuts have enjoyed for more than 2,000 years.

You are wondering what kind of exotic, ill-tasting grub do these Hunza people eat? It may sound very strange to you, actually everything the Hunzakuts eat is delectable to the western palate, and is readily available in the United States and Europe - at least if you shopping horizons do not begin and end at the supermarket.

Not only is the Hunza diet not exotic; there's really nothing terribly mysterious about its health-promoting qualities. Everything we know about food and health, gathered both from clinical studies and the observation of scientists who have traveled throughout the world observing dietary practices and their relationship to health, tells us that it is to be expected that the Hunza diet will go a long way towards improving the total health of anyone, anywhere. The Hunza story is only one of the more dramatic examples of the miraculous health produced by a diet of fresh, natural unprocessed and unadulterated food.

Are Hunza People that Healthy?

Maybe you're wondering: are the Hunzas really all that healthy? That was the question on the mind of cardiologists Dr. Paul D. White and Dr. Edward G. Toomey, who made the difficult trip up the mountain paths to Hunza, toting along with them a portable, battery-operated electrocardiograph. In the American Heart Journal for

December 1964, the doctors say they used the equipment to study 25 Hunza men, who were, "on fairly good evidence, between 90 and 110 years old." Blood pressure and cholesterol levels were also tested. They reported that not one of these men showed a single sign of coronary heart disease, high blood pressure or high cholesterol.

An optometrist, Dr. Allen E. Banik, also made the journey to Hunza to see himself if the people were as healthy as they were reputed to be, and published his report in Hunza Land (Whitethorn Publishing Co., 1960). "It wasn't long before I discovered that everything that I had read about perpetual life and health in this tiny country is true, "Dr. Banik declared."I examined the eyes of some of Hunza's oldest citizens and found them to be perfect."

Beyond more freedom from disease, the positive side of Hunza health has startled many observers. Dr. Banik, for example, relates that "many Hunza people are so strong that in the winter they exercise by breaking holes in the ice-covered streams and take a swim down under the ice." Other intrepid visitors who have been there report their amazement at seeing men 80, 90, and 100 years old repairing the always-crumbling rocky roads, and lifting large stones and boulders to repair the retaining walls around their terrace gardens. The oldsters think nothing of playing a competitive game of volleyball in the hot sun against men 50 years their junior, and even take part in wild games of polo that are so violent they would make an ice hockey fan shudder.

The energy and endurance of the Hunzakuts can probably be credited as much to what they don't eat as what they do eat. First of all, they don't eat a great deal of anything. The United States Department of Agriculture estimates that the average daily food intake for Americans of all ages amounts to 3,300 calories, with 100 grams of protein, 157 grams of fat and 380 grams of carbohydrates, In contrast, studies by Pakistani doctors show that adult males of Hunza consume a little more than 1.900 calories daily, with only 50 grams of protein, 36 grams of healthy fat, and 354 grams of carbohydrates. Both the **protein** and **fat** are **largely of vegetable origin** (Dr. Alexander Leaf, National Geographic, January, 1973).

That amounts to just half the protein, one-third the fat, but about the same amount of carbohydrates that we eat. Of course, the carbohydrate that the Hunzakuts eat is **undefined** or **complex carbohydrate** found in **fruits, vegetables** and **grains**, while we largely eat our carbohydrates in the form of nutrition like **white sugar** and **refined flour**.

Needless to say, the Hunzakuts eat **no processed food**. Everything is as fresh as it can possibly be. The only "processing" consists of **drying** some fresh fruits in the sun. No chemicals or artificial fertilizers are used in their gardens. In fact, it is against the law of Hunza to spray gardens with **pesticides.** Renee Taylor, in her book, Hunza Health Secrets (Prentice-Hall 1964) says that the Mir, or

127

ruler of Hunza, was recently instructed by Pakistani authorities to spray the orchards of Hunza with pesticide, to protect them from an expected invasion of insects. But the Hunzas would have none of it. They refused to use the **toxic pesticide**, and instead sprayed their trees with a mixture of **water** and **ashes**, which **adequately** protected the trees without poisoning the fruit and the entire environment. **In a word, the Hunzas eat as they live-organically.**

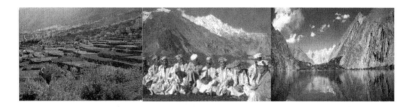

Apricots Are Hunza's Gold

Of all their organically grown food, perhaps their favorite, and one of their dietary mainstays, is the **apricot**. Apricot orchards are seen everywhere in Hunza, and a family's economic stability is measured by the number of trees they have under cultivation.

They eat their apricots **fresh in season**, and dry a great deal more in the sun for eating throughout the long cold winter. They puree the dried apricots and mix them with snow to make ice cream. Like their apricot jam, this ice cream needs no sugar because the apricots are so sweet naturally. But that is only the beginning.

The Hunzas cut the pits from the fruits, crack them, remove and eat the almond-like nuts. The women hand-grind these kernels with stone mortars, then squeeze the meal between a hand stone and a flat rock to **express the oil**. The oil is used in cooking, for fuel, as a salad dressing on fresh garden greens, and even as a **facial lotion** (Renee Taylor says Hunza women have beautiful complexions).

The Apricot Kernels Anti-Cancer Theory

Do these kernels have important protective powers, which in some way play an important role in the extraordinary health and longevity of the Hunza people? The **evidence** suggests they very well might. Cancer and arthritis are both very rare among the Taos (New Mexico) Pueblo Indians. Their traditional beverages are made from the group **kernels of cherries, peaches and apricots**.

Dr. Robert G. Houston told PREVENTION that he enjoyed this beverage when he was in New Mexico gathering material for a book dealing with blender shakes based on an Indian recipe. Into a glass of juice, he mixed freshly ground apricot kernels (1/4 of an ounce or two dozen kernels), which had been roasted for 10 minutes at 300 F. It is vitally important to roast the kernels first. Houston points out, "in order to ensure safety when you are using the pits in such quantities." Roasting destroys enzymes which could upset your stomach if you eat too many at on time. In any event the drink was so delicious that Houston kept having it daily. On the third day of drinking this concoction, Houston says that a funny thing happened. Two little benign skin growths on his arm, which formerly were pink, had turned brown. The next day, he noticed that the growths were black and shriveled. On the seventh morning, the smaller more recent growths had **vanished completely and the larger one about the size of a grain of rice had simply fallen off.**

Dr. Houston says that two of his friends have since tried the apricot shakes and report similar elimination of benign skin growths in one or two weeks. "Some foods, especially the kernels of certain fruits and grains, contain elements known as the nitrilosides also known as amygdalin or **Vitamin B 17**" says Dr. Ernst T. Krebs, Jr., biochemist and co-discoverer of Laetrile, a controversial cancer treatment (Laetrile is the proprietary name for one nitriloside). Nitrilosides, says Dr. Krebs, are non-toxic water-soluble, accessory food factors found in abundance in the **seeds** of almost **all fruits**. They are also found in over **100** other plants.

There are other common foods (all seeds), which provide a goodly supply of this protective factor, for example Hunzakuts eat in abundance **millet** and **buckwheat**. Lentils, beans and alfalfa, when sprouted, provide 50 times more nitrilosides than does the mature plant, Dr. Krebs points out. And the Hunzas, as you might expect, sprout all of their seeds, as well as using them in other ways. Since other essential protective elements are increased in the sprouting of such seeds, young sprouts are excellent foods, which give us more life-giving values than most of us realize.

Genesis 1:29

Then God said, *"I give you every seed-bearing plant on the face of the whole earth and every tree that has fruit with seed in it. They will be yours for food."*

Vitamin B 17

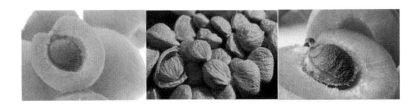

The Hunza people always crack open the kernel and eat the **seed.** The apricot seed contains Vitamin B17. Vitamin B17 is the **anticancer vitamin**. Some researchers have found that cancer and sickle cell anemia are caused by a **deficiency of vitamin B17.** Just as scurvy is caused by a deficiency of vitamin C, pernicious anemia is due to a deficiency of vitamin B12 and folic acid, and pellagra is caused by a deficiency of vitamin B3.

Vitamin B17 kills cancer cells without harming normal cells, **making it nature's chemotherapy**.

Various documents from the oldest civilisations such as Egypt at the time of the Pharaohs and from China 2,500 years before Christ mention the therapeutic use of derivatives of **bitter almonds**. Egyptian papyri from 5,000 years ago mention the use of "aqua amigdalorum" for the treatment of some **tumours** of the skin. But the systematised study of Vitamin B-17 really did not begin until the first half of the past century, when the chemist Bohn discovered in 1802 that during the distillation of the water from bitter almonds hydrocyanic acid was released. Soon many researchers became interested in analysing this extract, which they called AMYGDALIN (from amygdala = almond).

Vitamin B17 As a Preventative

According to Dr. Krebs, the basic concept is that sufficient daily B-17 may be obtained by following either of two suggestions:

First, eating all the B-17-containing food and seeds, but not eating more of the seeds by themselves than you would be eating if you ate them in the whole fruit. Example: if you eat **three apples** a day, **the seeds in the three apples are sufficient B-17**. You would never eat a pound of apple seeds.

Second, one peach or apricot kernel per 10 lbs. of body weight is believed to be more than sufficient as a normal safeguard in cancer prevention and chemotherapy help, although precise numbers may vary from person to person in accordance with individual metabolism and dietary habits. A 170-lb man, for example, might consume up to 17 apricots or peach kernels per day and receive a biologically reasonable amount of Vitamin B-17.

And two important notes: Certainly, you can consume too much of anything. Too many kernels or seeds, for example, can be expected to produce unpleasant side effects. **Too much is too much!**

High concentrations of B-17 are obtained by eating the natural foods in their raw or sprouting stage.

So how does B17 kill cancer cells?

Firstly, we need to understand that our bodies use several enzymes to perform many tasks. Our body has one particular enzyme called Rhodanese, which is found in large quantities throughout the body but **is not present wherever there are cancer cells.** Yet, wherever you find cancer in the body, you find another enzyme called Beta-Glucosidase. So, we have the enzyme Rhodanese found everywhere in the body except at the cancer cells, and we have the enzyme Beta-Glucosidase found in very large quantities only at the cancer cell but not found anywhere else in the body. If there is no cancer in the body there is no enzyme Beta-Glucosidase.

Now the following is what scares most people. You see Vitamin B17 is made up of 2 parts glucose, 1 part Hydrogen Cyanide and 1 part Benzaldehyde (analgesic/painkiller). So it is very important you understand the following:

When **B17** is introduced to the body, the enzyme called Rhodanese breaks it down. The Rhodanese breaks the Hydrogen Cyanide and Benzaldehyde down into 2 by-products, Thiocyanate and Benzoic acid, which are beneficial in **nourishing healthy cells** and forms the metabolic pool production for vitamin B12. Any excess of these by-products is expelled in normal fashion from the body via urine. Vitamin B17 passes through your body and does not last longer than 80 minutes inside your body as a result of the Rhodanese breaking it down. (Hydrogen Cyanide has been proven to be chemically inert and non-toxic when taken as food or refined pharmaceutical such as laetrile. Sugar has been shown to be 20 times more toxic than B17 - see good & bad cyanide).

AND HERE IS THE BEST PART:

When the B17 comes into contact with **cancer cells**, there is no Rhodanese to break it down and neutralize it but instead, only the enzyme Beta-Glucosidase is present in very large quantities. When B17 and Beta-Glucosidase come into contact with each other, a chemical reaction occurs and the Hydrogen Cyanide and Benzaldehyde

134

combine synergistically to produce a poison, which destroys and kills the cancer cells. This whole process is known as selective toxicity. Only the cancer cells are specifically targeted and destroyed. See the diagram below

Here is an illustration of how Vitamin B17 Kills Cancer. It has been proven to work by the some of the top cancer specialists in the world.

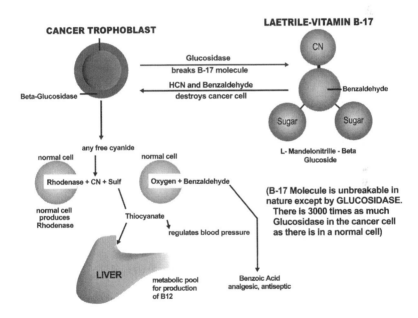

The best as you know is to have everything in moderation, and we have to apply this rule here. I would recommend you take up to 5 apricot kernels a day plus the amount of apple seeds you can find in 2-3 apples and have the variety of food that contains Vitamin B 17 like spinach, alfalfa, beans etc. In the chart below you can see the food that is the most rich in B 17. The best way is to have variety of recommended food every day, that way you get the most nutrients and heal, **alkalize** and **detox** your body as quick as possible.

Vitamin B17 and foods that contain it

Vitamin B17 or Laetrile appears in abundance in untamed nature. Because B17 is bitter to the taste, in man's attempt to improve tastes and flavors for his own pleasure, he has eliminated bitter substances like B17 by selection and crossbreeding.

As a general rule, many of the foods that have been domesticated still contain the vitamin B17 in that part not eaten by modern man, such as the seeds in apricots as you know already.

Listed below is an evaluation of some of the more common foods. Keep in mind that these are averages only and that specimens vary widely depending on variety, locale, soil, and climate.

All fruits that are mentioned below should be organically grown and ripe.

Foods	Low content (below 100 mgs nitriloside per 100 grams food)	Medium content (above 100 mgs nitriloside per 100 grams food)	High content (above 100 mgs nitriloside per 100 grams food)
Fruits	Domestic blackberry, market cranberry	Boysenberry, currant, elderberry (medium to high), gooseberry, huckleberry, loganberry, mulberry, quince, raspberry	Wild blackberry, choke cherry, wild crab-apple, Swedish (lignon) cranberry
Seeds		Buckwheat, flax, millet,	Apple seed, apricot seed, cherry seed, nectarine seed, peach seed, pear seeds, plum seed, prune seed, squash seeds
Beans	Black, black-eyed peas, garbanzo (low to medium), green pea, kidney (low to medium), U.S. lima, shell	Lentils, Burma lima, mung (medium to high)	Fava
Leaves	Beet tops, spinach, water cress		Alfalfa, eucalyptus,

Nuts (raw)	Cashew	Macadamia (medium to high)	Bitter almond
Sprouts		Alfalfa, fava, garbanzo, mung	Bamboo
Tubers	Sweet potato, yams		Cassava

Chapter 9

Detox & Purification Techniques

"Understanding is the first step to acceptance, and only with acceptance can there be recovery."

J.K. Rowling

Why is detoxification of your body important?

Toxic agents and substances are everywhere in our world. The food we eat, the air we breathe, the household cleaners we spray, and the electronics we use on a daily basis. However, toxic free radicals are formed in the human body too. Stress hormones, emotional disturbances, anxiety and negative emotions all create free radicals as well. Living without toxic build up is virtually impossible, which is why our body has built in mechanisms to deal with toxic overload. Crying, sweating, urination and defecation are all natural protocols employed by the body to rid itself of toxins.

Despite overwhelming advancements in medical care our society is sicker than ever. We may be living longer, but we're riddled with illness and disease. Nearly all sickness in industrialized countries is due to toxic build up in the body. Often times toxins bind to sex hormones or thyroid hormones, which slows metabolism, causing weight gain. Additionally, toxins are stored in fat cells, also contributing to excess weight. Cardiovascular disease, cancer, polycystic ovarian syndrome, infertility, gastroesophageal reflux disease, fatty liver, gallstones, osteoarthritis, stroke, lower back pain, headaches, carpal tunnel syndrome, dementia, asthma and depression are just some of the illnesses associated with obesity.

Because toxins affect both the structure and function of cells, they cause a myriad of health problems in their own right. Chronic fatigue, fibromyalgia, autoimmune disorders like multiple sclerosis and lupus, migraines, premature aging, digestive problems like constipation, diarrhoea or bloating, skin conditions, aches and pains, PMS and food allergies or intolerances are all the result of toxic build up in the body.

Detoxification is so important because it can literally reverse the symptoms of illness and change your life. There are many different types of detoxification protocols and it is important to find one that works well for you. The liver, small intestine, kidneys, and colon are the major organs involved in the body's detoxification system. However, when employing any type of cleanse (like a juice cleanse, liver and gallbladder cleanse, elimination diet, heavy metal cleanse, etc.) it is important to first cleanse the kidneys and colon, as these two eliminative organs are responsible for carrying toxic waste out of the body. If they aren't cleared of blockages, you can end up with even more toxic build up, as the toxins that are being expelled have nowhere to go. Herbal formulas are especially good at cleansing the kidneys. Colon hydrotherapy, enemas and Epsom salt cleanses are all excellent way to cleanse the colon.

As a nutritionist though, I feel compelled to reiterate that **juice cleansing** is an absolutely wonderful way to thoroughly cleanse your entire body. Juice cleansing regimens can help you to lose unwanted fat, boost your mental clarity, improve the state of your skin, regulate digestion, and, most important, **remove toxins** from your system, which is so critical in the case of chemotherapy or radiation. Because you do not have to chew and break down food, your digestive system is given a rest and allowed time to repair and rejuvenate. Juicing your food floods your body with **live enzymes** and an **abundance of antioxidants** that help not only neutralize free radicals but also strengthen and support the immune system, reduce blood pressure, improve sleep, concentration and memory, improve circulation and increase energy. Antioxidants even have anti-aging properties! They are literally a life-changing miracle food, and juice cleansing is an excellent way to inundate your system with them.

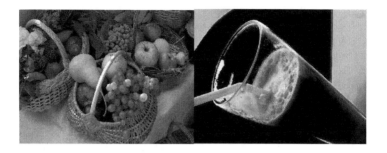

1. Alkalize your system by eliminating the food that contains too much acidity from your diet and include **Wheatgrass fresh juice** on its own or combined with other organically grown **fruit** or **vegetable** juices according to your taste. It is necessary to remove excess **acidity** and **toxic chemicals** from the body before health can be restored. To remove excess acidity from the tissues it is necessary to build up a reserve of alkalinity through an **alkaline (vegetarian) diet**, supplemented with **fresh fruit and vegetable juices** and **alkaline minerals**. Then this alkalinity must be moved around the body by any technique that works, such as exercise, massage, yoga, manual lymph drainage, etc. Vigorous **exercise** such as on the rebound mini-trampoline is reported to increase lymph flow by 15 to 30 times.

2. Avoid, at any cost, all dairy products including milk, cheese, yogurt, cream and ice cream with the exception of butter in small quantities. Include delicious versions of cereals and nuts drinks such as Almond Milk, Brown Rice Milk, Hazelnut Milk, Oat Milk, Quinoa Milk, etc.

3. The digestive system requires a rest periodically, even if just one day each week. Restricting the quantity of food consumed gives the system an opportunity to cleanse itself. The consumption of **fresh juices** made from **organically grown fruits and vegetables** during this time of reduced food consumption provides **alkalinity** to neutralize the acid wastes released from the tissues. It is important to understand that the doctors are not recommending "fasting" in the sense that you consume nothing but water. Rather they are recommending a liquid diet of fresh juices for a brief period (Diamond, pages 63, 341-42, 955).

4. Most people don't drink enough fluids and are chronically **dehydrated** without realizing. We usually tend to drink liquids when feeling thirsty and this is already a critical stage of the body by then. As a result, the kidneys are overworked. A lot of people think that the more fluid they drink the more the kidneys must work to remove it. However, what is difficult for kidneys is to remove waste. Removing fluid is easy for the kidneys. The reason for this is the "**concentration gradient**". When people drink half the necessary amount of fluid, then waste in the urine is twice as concentrated. It is concentrating the waste that is difficult for the kidneys, because the kidneys need to overcome osmotic pressure that wants to equalize concentrations on both sides of the membrane. Healthy kidneys can achieve a concentration gradient of about 3:1. If you drink twice as much fluid then the wastes are diluted by half, allowing the kidneys to remove twice as much

143

waste. **So drink more fluids and help the kidneys do their job.**

Up to 60% of the human body is water, the brain is composed of 70% water, and the lungs are nearly 90% water. Lean muscle tissue contains about 75% water by weight, body fat contains 10% water and bone has 22% water. About 83% of our blood is water, which helps digest our food, transport waste, and control body temperature. Each day humans must replace 2.4 liters of water, some through drinking and the rest taken by the body from the foods eaten.

Though as was mentioned above, please do not drink water less than 15 min before meals and not less than 40-45 min after meals.

5. An **alkaline condition** in the body increases zeta potential. Zeta potential is a measure of the electrical force that exists between atoms, molecules, particles, cells, etc., in a fluid. Zeta potential's strength determines the amount of nutrients and wastes that your blood and lymph can carry. Increasing the electrical force in the blood and lymph allows the fluid to dissolve and hold more nutrients, as a result releasing more waste. In this way, more nutrients can be carried throughout your body and **accumulated deposits of waste can be removed.** Aluminium (from food additives, cooking utensils, municipal drinking water, vaccines, drugs, etc.) destroys zeta potential.

Municipal (tap) drinking water contains chlorine. Chlorine has been used to disinfect our drinking water because it controls the growth of such unwelcome bacteria as Ecoli and Giardia. You have to be careful though when drinking tap water. Research has shown that long-term exposure to chlorine leads to the production of free radicals within the body. Free radicals as you know from above are carcinogenic, and cause tremendous damage to our cells.

The risk of developing cancer is 93% higher in people who drink or are otherwise exposed to chlorinated water.

How To Eliminate Chlorine in Water

- Consider a water purification system for your home. It will help to eliminate toxins before the water is used to cook, clean, shower and bathe.

- Use water filters in sinks and bathtubs. Water filters are an excellent way to ensure that your family is protected against the harmful effects of chlorine exposure.

- After you are exposed to chlorine, you should cleanse your body immediately. Use organic or all-natural soaps and detergents, as these are better for your skin. There are many kinds of soaps available that are not toxic.

Always drink purified water. Even better is oxygenated purified water, which provides added oxygen to your body.

6. Bile is an important avenue for detoxification of the body. It is a liquid produced by the **liver** and stored in the gallbladder until we eat a meal, and then it flows into the small intestine where it digests fats. Liver removes toxic chemicals from the blood, which flow out of the body via the bile and digestive tract. When the body produces more bile, the digestion improves and **more toxins** can be excreted via the bile. Inadequate bile flow allows toxins to build up in the body and results in liver disease, immune responses (allergies), skin problems, damaged arteries, arterial plaque, high blood pressure, chronic inflammation, arthritis, oedema (fluid build up), and cancer.

An **acid condition** in the body **causes bile to thicken**, eventually resulting in gallstones. Again you see the importance of an alkaline condition in the body, resulting in the bile to flow. Foods that help **increase bile** production and flow include **artichoke, lecithin, turmeric, and the herb milk thistle**.

Adequate bile is also needed for the body to digest and absorb fat-soluble vitamins and essential fatty acids.

7. Read the ingredients of all products you buy and make sure there are **no** sugar, soy, soybean oil, canola oil, bleached or unbleached wheat flower, soy flower, high fructose corn syrup (HFCS), corn syrup, trans fat, MSG, Aspartame, artificial sweeteners or dairy products.

8. Cook food using only coconut oil or virgin olive oil. Steam food rather than boiling when possible.

9. Steam bath and sauna are very helpful ways to purify the body through excessive sweating which removes toxic chemicals, and also because "**cancer cells die at temperatures between 104°F to 105.8°F** "(Diamond, page 996), whereas healthy cells survive.

Organic foods

As you noticed earlier in my book I emphasized the benefit of selecting organically grown foods. The explanation of this recommendation is quite simple. I would like you to understand in more detail the process of growing organic products and as a result the difference between organic products and conventional products.

Conventional vs. organic farming

The word "organic" refers to the way farmers grow and process agricultural products, such as fruits, vegetables, grains, fish, meat, etc. Organic farming practices are designed to encourage soil and water conservation and reduce pollution. Farmers who grow organic produce and meat don't use conventional methods to fertilize, control weeds or prevent livestock disease. For example, rather than using chemical weed killers, organic farmers may conduct more sophisticated crop rotations and spread mulch or manure to keep weeds at bay.

Here are some key differences between conventional farming and organic farming:

Conventional	Organic
Apply chemical fertilizers to promote plant growth.	Apply natural fertilizers, such as manure or compost, to feed soil and plants.
Spray synthetic insecticides to reduce pests and disease.	Spray pesticides from natural sources; use beneficial insects and birds, mating disruption or traps to reduce pests and disease.
Use synthetic herbicides to manage weeds.	Use environmentally generated plant-killing compounds; rotate crops, till, hand weed or mulch to manage weeds.
Give animals antibiotics, growth hormones and medications to prevent disease and spur growth.	Give animals organic feed and allow them access to the outdoors. Use preventive measures — such as rotational grazing, a balanced diet and clean housing — to help minimize disease.

The choice is yours! We are helping your body to detoxify, nourish, strength and heal itself with all available sources, and the right decision here is quite obvious.

More on Detoxification

Take Artichoke supplements or eat as a vegetable.

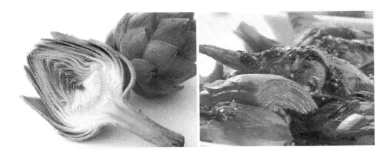

The Globe Artichoke is much valued at the table as a nutritious vegetable, but it is also an important aid to digestion and has been used to prevent arteriosclerosis. Artichoke extracts are said to be helpful for **kidney**, **gallbladder** and **liver insufficiency**, postoperative anaemia; and in some countries, Artichoke is considered a fine aphrodisiac.

Beneficial Uses:

The Artichoke has been used as an aid to good digestion and a means to improve **liver health**. Due to its cynarin content, it stimulates the **flow of bile from the liver into the intestines**, assisting the body in blood fat metabolism. Artichoke extracts are commercially available in Germany and Switzerland as a remedy for indigestion and in the U. K. as over-the counter digestive supplements. The **cynarin compound**, which is found in the leaves, stimulates the **gallbladder** and **improves liver function**. Artichoke has been used traditionally and in alternative medicine for treating dyspepsia, indigestion, nausea, flatulence, as well as liver and gallbladder ailments, including jaundice and hepatitis.

By helping the body to metabolize blood fat, the cynarin content in Artichoke is also believed to reduce blood lipids, serum cholesterol and triglyceride levels and is thought to be helpful in controlling arteriosclerosis.

In 2008, U.K. research confirmed that Artichoke leaf extract could reduce cholesterol levels in healthy adults. The studies determined that when Artichoke leaf extract was administered to otherwise healthy adults with raised cholesterol, levels dropped 6%.

Highly nutritious Artichoke is considered a diuretic, **promoting the flow of urine and appears to be effective in improving kidney function.** Artichoke is also frequently used to relieve **excess water weight** and peripheral oedema, a condition in which the peripheral body tissues contain an excessive amount of tissue fluid.

Other qualities attributed to Artichoke use include hypoglycaemic activity that may assist in **lowering blood glucose levels**. Artichoke has had traditional uses in USA and Spain for treating **diabetes**.

It is one of the world's oldest cultivated vegetables, grown by the Greeks and Romans at the height of their power and used for **food** and **medicine**. In ancient Greek mythology, the god Zeus was said to love the Globe Artichoke, which gave rise to its nickname "Vegetable of the Gods."

Artichoke **leaves**, **flower heads** and **root** are used **medicinally**, and the leaves are cut just before flowering for use fresh or dried in liquid extracts, syrups and capsules. The French have long used Artichoke juice as a **liver tonic**, because of the herb's abilities to **break down fat** and improve **bile flow**.

Artichoke leaves contain a wide number of active constituents, including **cynarin** and **cholorogenic acid, flavonoids**, protein, **amino acids, calcium, phosphorus, potassium, folic acid, vitamin C, niacin, thiamine**, trace minerals and carotenoids.

Recommended Dosage:
Take two (2) capsules, two (2) times each day with water at mealtimes.

Contraindications:

Artichoke is not recommended for those who are allergic to Artichokes or other members of the *composites* (daisy) family. At the recommended amount and according to the German Commission E Monograph, there are no known side effects or drug interactions. **Those who have any obstruction of the bile duct (gallstones) should not take Artichoke.**

I would highly recommend, if you have the means and time to invest in a treatment of your body, mind and spirit by visiting, for a week or two, the Optimum Health Institute (OHI).

They have two locations, one in Texas and the other one in San Diego, California. OHI can offer you excellent programs for detoxification, cleansing and body nourishment as well as your mind and spirit.

OHI HOLISTIC HEALING PROGRAM:

In Optimum Health Institute's holistic healing program, participants cleanse and nourish the body with **diet**, juicing, fasting, and exercise; quiet and focus the mind with journaling and meditation; and renew and awaken the spirit with study, prayer and celebration.

Cleansing and Nourishing Your Body:

Your body is self-healing. When given the proper tools to work with, it can restore itself to its natural balance.

Practiced for many centuries around the world, detoxification is the process of cleansing the body to promote healing and longevity. To help your body cleanse and restore itself, OHI provides:

- **Wheatgrass juice** to cleanse cells and purify blood
- **Enemas** and **wheatgrass implants** to cleanse the colon
- **Gentle exercise** to cleanse the lymphatic system

OHI contracts with qualified professionals to make optional services available to you. These services supplement the core OHI holistic healing program:

- **Massages and spa treatments** to remove congestion and release tension
- **Colon hydrotherapy** to eliminate toxins
- **Chiropractic** care to reduce structural or nerve pain

Contact information:

Optimum Health Institute of San Diego

6970 Central Avenue
Lemon Grove, CA 91945

Call to make a reservation

(800) 993-4325
(619) 464-3346

Optimum Health Institute of Austin

265 Cedar Lane
Cedar Creek, TX 78612

Call to make a reservation

(800) 993-4325
(512) 303-4817

Website: http://www.optimumhealth.org

Chapter 10

Historically Proven Herbal Recipes To Kill Cancer Cells

The Hoxsey Therapy

"Inaction breeds doubt and fear. Action breeds confidence and courage. If you want to conquer fear, do not sit home and think about it. Go out and get busy."

Dale Carnegie

Herbal treatments are documented as the oldest type of approach to cancer and have been **used with success for thousands of years by indigenous people all around the world.**

In recent years, modern science has proven that many herbs do, in fact, have **cancer-fighting properties**. They have been shown to support the body's **immune system**, improve **blood circulation**, strengthen the functioning of major organs, and enhance the efficient **elimination of toxins**, among other things. **They can act very much like a potent drug as well.** For instance, some herbs have direct

155

cytotoxic effects on the cancer cells themselves, while not harming other cells of the body. Other herbs have been shown to inhibit a tumor's ability to produce **new blood vessels** to feed itself, thereby strangling the tumor's system of nourishment. And still other herbs have **anti-microbial properties**. Thus, herbs are often referred to as "nature's medicine" and the **Hoxsey therapy for cancer is a wonderful example of this.**

The Hoxsey therapy was the first widely used alternative non-toxic treatment for cancer in the modern United States. Still obtainable today, it is a treatment that consists of an herbal topical salve, an herbal topical powder, and an herbal internal tonic. Though many people have never heard of it, this treatment approach was very successful and was actually used by tens of thousands of Americans in the early to mid-1900s. Around 1953, at the height of the Hoxsey therapy, the main Hoxsey clinic in Dallas, Texas had 12,000 patients and was the largest private cancer center in the world. There were also subsidiary clinics in 17 other states.

History

Harry Hoxsey, an American born in 1901-1974, was the person responsible for the widespread use of the Hoxsey therapy for cancer. The herbal remedy had been passed down to Harry by his great-grandfather, John Hoxsey. It was John Hoxsey, a horse breeder in Illinois, who developed the herbal remedy. In 1840 Harry's great-grandfather John had a stallion that was expected to die as a result of having developed a cancerous lesion on its leg. This horse had been one of John's favorites, so when the horse had to be put out to pasture, he kept an eye on it. He noticed that the horse exhibited atypical behavior by grazing primarily on one clump of shrubs and flowering plants. He also noticed that the horse's cancer completely healed after a number of months and the stallion made a full recovery.

Curious about his horse's amazing return to health, John picked samples from the plants on which the stallion had been grazing. Through experimentation, he developed an herbal tonic, salve, and powder from them. Some think John Hoxsey may have also gotten input from some of the local Native Americans about the use of these plants. He then started using these remedies to treat other horses suffering from external cancers or other types of lesions. John's herbal mixture proved to be quite successful, and word spread quickly until horse breeders were bringing their horses to him from as far away as Indiana and Kentucky.

John Hoxsey's herbal mixtures were eventually passed down to Harry's father, a veterinarian. Harry's father used the herbal remedies to treat animals with cancer and other conditions. But he started to quietly use the herbal treatments to help humans with cancer as well.

When Harry was eight years old, he began assisting his father in administering these treatments to some of the local people. These were generally people who had no other hope for recovery, and the Hoxsey remedies were having success. Just before his father's death, Harry, the youngest in a family of 12 children, was entrusted with the secrets of how to prepare the remedies and was given the responsibility to carry on the family's healing tradition.

The Hoxsey therapy was mostly known for its success with external tumors on the surface of the body. People with external cancers were treated with an herbal paste applied directly onto the tumor and given a liquid herbal tonic to drink as well. People with **internal cancer** that showed no external signs were just given the Hoxsey's tonic. Certain dietary changes were also recommended to patients in general, along with a few nutritional supplements.

The Hoxsey Tonic ingredients:

RED CLOVER BLOSSOM
LICORICE ROOT
BUCKTHORN BARK
BURDOCK ROOT
STILLINGIA ROOT
POKE ROOT
BARBERRY ROOT
OREGON GRAPE ROOT
CASCARA SAGRADA BARK
PRICKLY ASH BARK
WILD INDIGO ROOT
SEA KELP
POTASSIUM IODIDE

Though it was not proven at the time, botanists have since found all of the herbs in the Hoxsey tonic to have various anti-cancer properties. And the external salve contains bloodroot, which has been used by Native Americans to treat cancer for centuries.

Ranch wife Della Mae Nelson had uterine cancer that had been extensively treated with twenty units of X-ray and thirty-six hours of radium. She was so badly burned from the radiation that she couldn't even pull a sheet over her body for a year after. Wasted to eighty-six pounds, she was bleeding internally, so severely impaired that she had to learn to walk all over again. Then the cancer recurred.

When Della Mae's cancer recurred, her conventional doctors told the family there was nothing more they could do for her. Against her daughter's wishes, Della Mae then sought treatment at the Hoxsey clinic in Dallas. She, too, completely recovered from her cancer as a result of the Hoxsey therapy. (Della Mae Nelson died about 50 years later, in 1997, at the age of ninety-nine. She had outlived most of the conventional doctors and nurses that had treated her).

All of the Hoxsey clinics admitted and treated any cancer patient who came to them, even *those that could not pay*. Ausubel's book documents numerous times when Hoxsey exhibited generosity to his patients above and beyond the call of duty, including fully treating people who had used up their last dime on bus fare to get to the clinic. Many times Hoxsey then drove them to a local place where they could stay. In reality, Hoxsey was following the advice his father had given him when he handed the responsibility of the family remedies over. His father said:

"Now you have the power to heal the sick and save lives. What I've managed to do in a tiny part of this state, you can do all over the country, all over the world. I've cured hundreds of people. You can cure thousands, tens of thousands.

But it's not only a gift, son; it's a trust and a great responsibility. Abe Lincoln once said God must have loved the common people because he made so many of them. We're common, ordinary people. You must never refuse to treat anybody because he can't pay. Promise me that!"

In 1954, an independent group of 10 doctors from various parts of the United States made a point of investigating Hoxsey's clinic in Dallas. After the two-day inspection, which included examining hundreds of case histories and talking to patients and ex-patients, this independent group of physicians made a stunning public conclusion. **They reported that the Hoxsey clinic is successfully treating pathologically proven cases of cancer, both internal and external, without the use of surgery, radium or x-ray.**

Accepting the standard yardstick of cases that have remained symptom- free in excess of five to six years after treatment, established by medical authorities, we have seen sufficient cases to warrant such a conclusion. Some of those presented before us have been free of symptoms as long as twenty-four years, and the physical evidence indicates that they are all enjoying exceptional health at this

160

time.

Doctors CONCLUSION:

We as a Committee feel that the Hoxsey treatment is superior to such conventional methods of treatment as x-ray, radium, and surgery.

Current Hoxsey Therapy

The Bio-Medical Center in Tijuana continues to operate and administer the Hoxsey therapy. Information below indicates how to contact this treatment center.

Contact information:

BIOMEDICAL CENTER

Location: 3170 General Ferreira Col. Juarez - Tijuana, Baja California - 22150 MEXICO

Mailing address: PO box 433654 - San Isidro, CA 92143 - 3654

Telephone: (011-52664) 684-90-11 - Fax: (011-52664) 684-97-44

Email: bmed@bc.cablemas.com

It is not as expensive as many therapies - it costs only $3500 for the therapy no matter how long it takes, with 30% due at the first appointment.

In addition to the Hoxsey treatment, comprised of a liquid elixir containing a mixture of herbs and several topical salves, the clinic may also use other supplements, diet, nutrition, and chelation therapy. They treat most types of malignancies, but it is said to be especially effective with skin cancer (including melanoma), breast cancer, and has been successful with some recurrent cancers and even with patients who've had radiation and/or chemotherapy.

Essiac Tea

*"Put **LOVE** first. Entertain thoughts that give life. And when a thought or resentment, or hurt, or fear comes your way, have another thought that is more powerful – a thought that is **LOVE**"*

Mary Morrissey

Essiac Tea is a long proven method of curing cancer. It dates back to the 1920s and before.

What is the history of the discovery and use of Essiac and Flor Essence as complementary or alternative treatments for cancer?

Essiac was created by a Canadian nurse called Renee Caisse. She named the remedy after herself - Essiac is her surname spelled backwards. Other names for Essiac include 'Flor essence' and 'tea of life'. Renee Caisse first began to promote Essiac as a cancer treatment in the 1920s. Today, Essiac and Flor Essence may be sold as herbal supplements as long as they do not claim to treat or cure cancer.

- In 1922, a breast cancer patient gave the Essiac formula to the nurse and said it had cured her disease. The patient said the formula came from an Ontario Ojibwa Native American medicine man.

- In 1934, the nurse opened a cancer clinic in Ontario and gave Essiac to patients free of charge. In 1938, the Royal Cancer Commission of Canada visited the clinic but found little evidence that Essiac was effective. The nurse closed the clinic in 1942 but continued to give Essiac to patients until the late 1970s.

- Between 1959 and the late 1970s, the nurse worked with an American doctor to study Essiac in the laboratory and in people and to promote its use. They also created the formula now called Flor Essence. The results of their studies were not reported in any peer-reviewed scientific journals. Most scientific journals have experts who review research reports before they are published, to make sure that the evidence and conclusions are sound. Studies published in peer-reviewed scientific journals are considered to be better evidence.

In the 1980s, companies making Essiac-like products began to sell the mixtures as health tonics. Because these companies did not make claims that it would treat or cure certain diseases, Essiac did not come under laws that regulate it as a drug.

While the basic components of Essiac are well known, the exact proportions of the herbs in Essiac are the matter of much speculation. The cancer patient should be far more concerned with the quality of the herbs, and the quality of the processing, than with the exact formula. Some brands have 4, 6 or 8 herbs (e.g. Flor-Essence has 8 herbs). The extra herbs won't hurt, and may be of some help. But again, the quality of the herbs, and the quality of the processing, is the most important issue.

It should be mentioned that it is the **Sheep Sorrel** that is the **main cancer-killing herb** in Essiac. Sheep Sorrel has been known about for over a hundred years as a **cancer-fighting herb**.

The Four Main Essiac Tea Ingredients:

Burdock Root

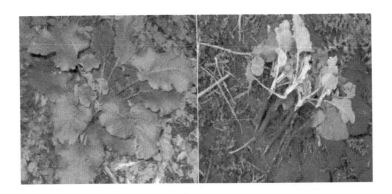

Burdock root has been known to be an effective blood purifier for centuries now. Its seeds contain oil that is eliminated through sweating; taking poisons and toxins with it and it also helps heal some skin problems. Burdock root also contains niacin, which is known for ridding the body of toxins, like those absorbed through radiation. Burdock root also is been known to dissolve kidney stones, as well as provide support for the bladder and liver. Minerals such as iron are abundant in this root. Studies have also shown that burdock can help shrink tumors or prevent it from growing. This property of Burdock root that prevents mutations is called the "B factor". The Japanese, who also use Burdock root in medicine, discovered this. The World Health Organization has also reported that Burdock is a potential treatment for HIV because it appears to be active against the virus. The extract form of Burdock root reportedly demonstrated strong anti-cancer activity against leukemia. Burdock is also used in another herbal cancer treatment you read about above which is **Hoxsey cancer treatment**. Check out this page to read more about burdock root benefits.

Sheep Sorrel

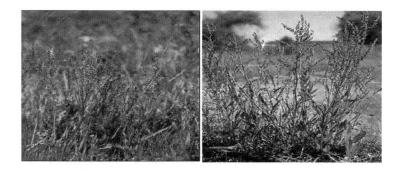

Sheep sorrel, when taken in different forms, yields different results. As a cool drink, it may lower your temperature if you have a fever. When taken as a tea, it is good for stomach pains and diarrhea. It could also be gargled, to alleviate sore throats. Its astringent properties also have been known to stop internal or external bleeding although it is recommended that you seek medical attention immediately instead of self-medicating with sheep sorrel.

Since sheep sorrel is high in antioxidants, it helps to protect cells from damage due to normal cell metabolism and/or destruction. Aside from having anti-tumor properties, it also appears to be an antiseptic and antibacterial. Some studies show strong evidence that this shrinks tumors in humans, while the other uses were mostly tested on mice. People suffering from arthritis can also find use for this as it has anti-inflammatory properties as well. Like fruits and vegetables, sheep sorrel contains many vitamins and minerals that could alleviate pains due to stress, fatigue, and other aches.

Its uses are related to the circulatory system, indicating that those who are suffering imbalances of this nature can benefit from this herb. Some less popular theories even claim that it has anti-angiogenesis properties. That basically means this herb may have the power to cut off the main energy source of tumors. This avenue of treatment is currently being studied as another way to cure cancer.

Slippery Elm Bark

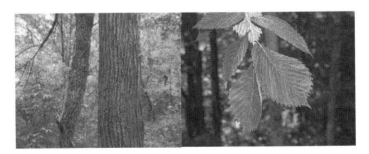

Before it was discovered for its medicinal purposes, this tree was made into houses, canoes, baskets and more. Soldiers relied on this as their food source to help them survive when lost at war.

The inner bark of this tree is mostly used for its soothing effects. In fact, it is considered safe enough for infants as well as pregnant women and the elderly. The soothing effects stem from its high mucilage content. Mucilage serves to strengthen and heal tissues. Before a tissue heals, it has to be soothed and stabilized from any prior irritation. Organs of the body that benefit most from this are the lungs, intestines and urinary tracts. It is a go-to food when one can barely ingest anything and is even as nutritious as oats. It's an excellent source of calcium, which is good for the nervous system and emotional wellbeing. A constituent called tannins makes this herb an astringent as well. When made into a paste, it can sooth wounds, burns, boils and other inflamed or painful surfaces. It is also reportedly used for drawing out the poison from a bullet wound.

Turkey Rhubarb Root

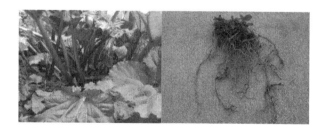

The name Turkey Rhubarb came to be from its early days as an export of China. This was mainly used for two cases: diarrhea and constipation. Smaller doses would help cease the sometimes-involuntary expulsion of waste, as larger doses were administered to help alleviate constipation.

It is a popular ingredient in many Chinese medicinal recipes. It also reportedly improves symptoms of kidney failure. It is an anti-tumor, anti-inflammatory, anti-bacterial and is more palatable than its counterpart, garden rhubarb root.

Turkish rhubarb is one of the most-discussed Essiac tea ingredients.

Essiac Tea Benefits: Primary Actions

Essiac tea's primary actions are to remove heavy metals, detoxify the body, restore energy levels, and rebuild the immune system. After this occurs, the body is restored to a level to where it is able to better defeat an illness or disease state *using its own resources*.

Everyone comes in contact with viruses and bacteria all the time, and everyone is susceptible to developing health problems. *People only get sick because their body's immune system FAILS to fight off the illness or infection.*

Therefore if the immune system is boosted, many illnesses and diseases can be eradicated WITH NO DRUGS. Essiac tea benefits the immune system more than any other substance we know of.

Here are some ESSIAC TEA benefits that have been reported and observed in research performed by Rene Caisse and Dr. Charles Brusch at the Brusch Medical Research Center.

Essiac Tea...

1. Prevents the buildup of excess fatty deposits in artery walls, heart, kidney and liver.

2. Regulates cholesterol levels by transforming sugar and fat into energy.

3. Destroys parasites in the digestive system and throughout the body.

4. Counteracts the effects of aluminum, lead and mercury poisoning.

5. Strengthens and improves the functioning of muscles, organs and tissues.

6. Makes bones, joints, ligaments, lungs, and membranes strong and flexible, and therefore less vulnerable to stress or stress injuries.

7. Nourishes and stimulates the brain and nervous system.

8. Promotes the absorption of fluids in the tissues.

9. Removes toxic accumulations in the fat, lymph, bone marrow, bladder, and alimentary canals.

10. Neutralizes acids, absorbs toxins in the bowel, and eliminates both.

11. Clears the respiratory channels by dissolving and expelling mucus.

12. Relieves the liver of its burden of detoxification by converting fatty toxins into water-soluble substances that can then be easily eliminated through the kidneys.

13. Assists the liver to produce lecithin, which forms part of the myelin sheath, a white fatty material that encloses nerve fibers.

14. Reduces, perhaps eliminates, heavy metal deposits in tissues (especially those surrounding the joints) to reduce inflammation and stiffness.

15. Improves the functions of the pancreas and spleen by increasing the effectiveness of insulin.

16. Purifies the blood.

17. Increases red cell production, and keeps them from rupturing.

18. Increases the body's ability to utilize oxygen by raising the oxygen level in the tissue cells.

19. Maintains the balance between potassium and sodium within the body so that the fluid inside and outside each cell is regulated; in this way, cells are nourished with nutrients and are also cleansed properly.

20. Converts calcium and potassium oxalates into a harmless form by making them solvent in the urine. Regulates the amount of oxalic acid delivered to the kidneys, thus reducing the risk of stone formation in the gall bladder, kidneys, or urinary tract.

21. Protects against toxins entering the brain.

22. Protects the body against radiation and X-rays.

23. Relieves pain.

24. Speeds up wound healing by regenerating the damaged area.

25. Increases the production of antibodies like lymphocytes and T-cells in the thymus gland, which is the defender of our immune system.

26. Protects the cells against free radicals.

27. Increases the appetite for healthful foods.

28. Decreases sugar cravings due to better blood sugar control.

29. Increases energy available.

30. Boosts mood and leads to an improved sense of well being.

Testimonials from cancer patients who achieved complete remission or considerable improvement using **Essiac** are obtainable from Elaine Alexander. These remarkable letters document cases of the last fifteen years and encompass **many types of cancer, including pancreatic, breast, and ovarian cancer; cancers of the esophagus, bile ducts, bladder, and bones; and lymphoma and metastatic melanoma.**

Muriel Peters of Creston, British Columbia, one of the people who wrote to Elaine Alexander to describe her experience with Essiac, was diagnosed in 1981 with a malignant tumor the size of an orange on her coccyx, the triangular bone at the base of the spine. She underwent surgery a week later. The surgeons told her, "We got it all," but according to Muriel, "By the time they had found the tumor, it had begun to flare up the spine among the nerve endings, so they could not cut there." She had twenty-nine radiation treatments following the surgery. In September 1982, sensing numbness in her lower abdominal area, she went to the Cancer Clinic in Vancouver and was told by a head surgeon that the tumor had spread to her spine and was inoperable, and nothing more could be done.

When her brother-in-law mentioned a man with cancer who had been given three months to live but was cured "somewhere down South," Muriel Peters followed up the lead. One month later, she visited the Bio-Medical Center in Tijuana, Mexico, and began the Hoxsey herbal therapy. Within three months, sensation returned to her lower abdomen, but this was followed by "three months of excruciating pain which no pills could relieve." She then began taking Essiac in liquid form, which she obtained from the Resperin Corporation through her doctor. After twelve days, the pain subsided. "From then on I was on my way up."

For the next year and a half, Muriel took Essiac daily. She also remained on the Hoxsey regimen, which consisted of an herbal tonic, vitamin supplements, and a special diet stressing fresh vegetables, greens, and fruits. "I felt the two complemented each other," Muriel explains. "Without the diet and the vitamins, I really doubt if either of the tonics would have been quite enough. The body has to rebuild

174

what the cancer has broken down; therefore healthy foods are needed by the body to reconstruct itself."

About a year after she started her dual program, Muriel returned for tests to the Vancouver Cancer Clinic. Incredulous, the attending doctor told her, "For reasons unknown there have been notable changes in your body."

"When the doctor left the room," recalls Muriel, "the attending nurse asked me what I was doing to bring about these changes, and I only said, 'I'm on a diet and vitamins.' The nurse asked, 'On your own?' I replied, 'No, by doctors directing.' She then said, 'Well, as long as you're not going to Mexican quacks, as many are doing.'"

A complete medical checkup in September 1989 found Muriel Peters cancer-free and in excellent health. At sixty-eight, she reported, "I'm the healthiest person in British Columbia. I love life and living.... I have learned what life is all about." X-rays and blood tests in January 1991 confirmed her to be in complete remission, nine years after she was diagnosed with inoperable, **"hopeless" cancer.**

Chapter 11

The connection between your Mind, Body and Emotions

*"The **Mind** in itself and in its own place can make a hell out of **Heaven** or a **Heaven** out of hell"*

John Milton

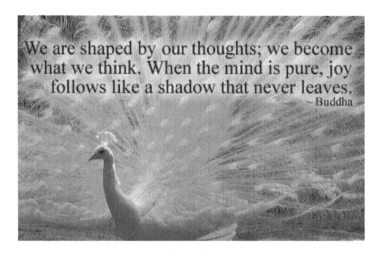

We are shaped by our thoughts; we become what we think. When the mind is pure, joy follows like a shadow that never leaves.
~ Buddha

Legendary psychologist and Holocaust-survivor Viktor Frankl once wrote, "Everything can be taken from a person but one thing: the last of human freedoms - to choose one's attitudes in any given set of circumstances, **to choose one's** own way." Frankl was right. **Attitude is a personal choice**. You could be faced with a thousand problems, many or most over which you have absolutely no control. However, there is always one thing you are in complete and absolute control of and that is your **own attitude** and therefore your actions!

Attitude is the composite of **your thoughts, feelings, emotions** and **actions**. Your **conscious mind** controls **feelings** and ultimately dictates whether your feelings will be **positive** or **negative** by your **choice of thoughts**, then your body displays those choices through **action** and **behavior.**

Attitude is actually a **creative cycle** that begins with your **choice of thoughts**. You **do** choose your thoughts and that choice is where your attitude originates. As you internalize ideas or become emotionally involved with your thoughts, you create the second stage in forming an attitude; you move your entire being - mind and body - into a new "vibration." Your conscious awareness of this vibration is referred to as "feelings". Your feelings are then expressed in actions or behaviors that produce the various results in your life.

Positive results are always the effect of a **positive attitude**.

Attitude and results are inseparable.

Simply stated, if you think in **negative terms**, you will get **negative results**; if you think in **positive terms** you will achieve **positive results**. Ralph Waldo Emerson reiterated that same point when he said, "**A person is what they think about all day long.**" The results you achieve in life are nothing more than an expression of your **thoughts, feelings**, and **actions**.

Winning and **losing** are opposite sides of the same coin - and that coin *is attitude.* There are many things wrong in this world; unfortunately that is all some people are able to see. Those who view the world in this light are often unhappy and somewhat cynical. Usually, their life is one of lack and limitation and it almost appears as if they move from one bad experience to another. I know people who are like this and I'm certain you do as well. It would appear as if they were born with a streak of bad luck and it has followed them around their whole life. These individuals are quick to **blame circumstances** or other **people** for their problems, rather than accepting **responsibility** for their life and their **attitude.**

Conversely, there are others who are forever winning and living the good life. They are the real movers and shakers who make things happen. They seem to go from one major accomplishment to another. They're in control of their life; they know where they are going and **know they will get**

there. They are the **real winners** in life and their wins are a matter of their **choice**.

Let's speaks about worries and stress. Of course you are worried and I completely understand it. Something I would like you to know is that **stress affects blood flow** within the body. Not everybody knows about this connection, otherwise people would pay more attention to their reactions and attitude. When the body becomes stressed, it channels more blood to the muscles of the arms and legs, causing less blood to go to the stomach. As a result, food is more slowly digested and instead remains in the stomach for longer periods of time. **Undigested food** is one of the primary causes of **acid** reflux as the food pushes up against the top of the stomach, opening a valve called the lower esophageal sphincter. When undigested food causes this sphincter to open, this allows acid to reflux back up from the stomach into the esophagus. This is one way in which increased stress can cause acid reflux.

We saw in earlier chapters how dangerous an acidic body environment is for us. Imagine how bad it is for the body if people eat acidic food on top of being stressed. Even if do everything else do make your body more alkaline and at the same time you are stressed and worried, the body will still produce dangerous acidity. If you stop and just think about your inner feelings, emotions, attitude to life you realize that it is only **you** who decides how to react to certain circumstances and what an attitude towards life to have.

You are a Master of your own choice of emotions, thought, feelings and actions!

Think about this...

During the day average person have approximately sixty thousands thoughts, and guess what: 85% of them exactly the same ones they had the day before and even worse that a lot of them are negative.

You may have heard or read the expression in the Bible "Drink water from your own well". You saw above the percentage of water our body and brain contains. So what is the quality of our water are when we allow ourselves to think negative thoughts and emotions? No wonder why many of us feel constantly exhausted.

Worry drains us of our natural vitality and energy. If you have a bicycle and its tires are fully inflated it will take you to your destination, when a tire has a leak it will deflate eventually and interrupt the journey. The same analogy can be applied with worry; it only causes your precious mental energy and potential to leak away, just like air leaking out of a tire.

Again it is in your own hands to stop worrying and invest your precious energy to win your health back with the knowledge your mind is equipped now. You can enjoy inner peace that you are doing everything to give your blood cells the highest opportunity to do the best for you.

One of the good techniques for ridding the mind of worry and other negative, life-draining influences is when any negative thought comes to your mind as they do so to all of us, to say "thank you" to that one and to then replace it with a positive thought. It is a very simple technique known for centuries as our mind can only hold one thought at any one time. Using this technique, anyone can easily create a positive, creative mind set within a short period of time. It is one or the other: your mind controls you or you control your mind. You are the Master of your thoughts and only you can decide which one you allow to enter your precious Mind!

In reality, the quality of your thinking determines the quality of your life. A strong, disciplined mind, which anyone can cultivate through daily practice, leads to powerful actions and as a result positive and desirable change!

We must be grateful and appreciative for everything we have and how often we forget to express that thought. The more we are thankful to God and people surrounding us for all we have and experienced on this beautiful planet the more positive change we will attract to our life.

Your positive mind will be a huge help for your beloved blood cells as they will be able to perform in completely different mode and you will see the transformation.

When you wake up in the morning ask yourself a question: "How am I going to enjoy myself today?" Think about it and include something in your day that you love to do or perhaps always wanted to do and never had time.

Dorothea Brand once said, "*Act as if it were impossible to fail,*" and I challenge you to do so. By simply becoming aware that you can choose what to nourish your body with, concentrating on positive thoughts, emotions, being grateful and as a result acting in this focused way each and every day, you will achieve your goal. You have to decide right now what you are going to do with your body, as you are its Master, and with your thoughts and emotions - and take an action.

You have the power to choose what you give your body to work with, no matter what your circumstances are. That positive personal choice will allow your blood cells to do the best work for your entire body and you can win your precious Health back! You don't have to be a prisoner of your past instead you can become an Architect of your present and future!

God Bless You!

*"Yesterday is a **history**, tomorrow is a **mystery**, **today is a gift of God**, which is why we call it the present."*

Bill Keane

References:

Airola, Ph.D., Paavo, How to Get Well, Health Plus, Sherwood, Oregon, 1993.
Altschul, Aaron M. Proteins, Their Chemistry and Politics, Basic Books, New York, 1965.
Barefoot, Robert R. And Carl J. Reich, M.D., The Calcium Factor: The Scientific Secret of Health and Youth, Gilliland Printing Inc., Arkansas City, Kansas, 1996.
Binzel, M.D., Philip E., Alive and Well - One Doctor's Experience with Nutrition in the Treatment of Cancer Patients, American Media. Westlake Village, CA, 1994. "In my attempts to use nutritional therapy, which includes the use of Laetrile, in the treatment of cancer, I have often been confronted by the Food and Drug Administration and by the State Medical Board. I have fought and, through the grace of God, I have won."
Budwig, Dr. Johanna, Flax Oil As a True Aid Against Arthritis, Heart Infarction, Cancer and Other Diseases, Apple Publishing Company Ltd., Vancouver, 1996.

Day, Phillip, Cancer - Why We're Still Dying To Know The Truth, Credence Publications, PO Box 3, Tonbridge, Kent TN12 9ZY, United Kingdom.
Diamond, M.D., W. John, W. Lee Cowden, M.D. with Burton Goldberg, An Alternative Medicine Definitive Guide to Cancer, Future Medicine Publishing, Inc., Tiburon, California, 1997.
Erasmus, Ph.D., Udo, Fats that Heal, Fats that Kill, Alive Books, 1993.
Fife, N.D., Bruce, The Coconut Oil Miracle, Avery, New York, 2004.
Fuhrman, M.D., Joel, Eat To Live: The Revolutionary Formula for Fast and Sustained Weight Loss, Little Brown, 2003.
Gerson, M.D., Max, A Cancer Therapy - Results of Fifty Cases and The Cure of Advanced Cancer by Diet Therapy - A Summary of 30 Years of Clinical Experimentation, Gerson Institute, Binita, California, 1990.
Griffin, G. Edward, World Without Cancer, American Media, Westlake Village, California, 1997. Both the book and video can be purchased directly from the author.

Jochems, Ruth, Dr. Moerman's Anti-Cancer Diet, Avery Publishing Group Inc., Garden City Park, New York, 1990. In Holland the vegetarian diet promoted by Dr. Moerman has been recognized by the government as a legitimate treatment for cancer. Results indicate that Dr. Moerman's diet is more effective than standard cancer treatments.
Kelley, Dr. William Donald, Cancer: Curing the Incurable Without Surgery, Chemotherapy, or Radiation, 2001. Newly revised and updated information from Dr. Kelley.

Kendall, Roger V., Building Wellness with DMG - How a breakthrough nutrient gives cancer, autism & cardiovascular patients a second chance at health, Freedom Press, 2003.

Lappe, Frances Moore, Diet for a Small Planet, Ballantine Books, New York, 1992. This book explains the principle of protein complementarity that is the basis of the vegetarian diet. By combining a grain and a legume you produce a protein that is as good as animal protein. Examples include: rice and lentils (rice and dahl - India), corn and beans (Mexico), chick peas and wheat (falafel sandwich - Middle East). This famous bread recipe takes full advantage of protein complementarity: "Take wheat and barley, beans and lentils, millet and spelt; put them in a storage jar and use them to make bread for yourself." - Ezekiel 4:9. A high protein plant diet provides twice the vitamins and minerals of a meat diet, and vastly more fiber, phyto-nutrients, and other required nutrients.

McDaniel, T.C., Disease Reprieve, Xlibris Corporation, 1999. Understanding zeta potential and human health.

McTaggart, Lynne, What Doctors Don't Tell You, First Avon Books, New York, 1998.

Montignac, Michel, Eat Yourself Slim, Alex & Lucas Publishing, 2004.

Pierce, N.D., Carson E., What I Would Do If I Had Cancer Again, 1996.

Robbins, John, Reclaiming Our Health, H J Kramer Inc., Tiburon, California, 1998.

Sharma, M.D., Hari, Freedom from Disease, Veda Publishing, Toronto, Ontario, 1993.

Sharma, M.D., Hari, et al, The Answer To Cancer Is Never Giving It A Chance to Start, Select Books, New York, 2002.

Taylor, Ross, with forward by Olivia Newton-John, Living Simply With Cancer, Cancer Support Association, Perth, Western Australia, 1998.

Whang, Sang, Reverse Aging, Siloam Enterprise, Inc., Englewood Cliffs, NJ, 1994.

Young, M.D., Robert O., The pH Miracle: Balance Your Diet; Reclaim Your Health, Wellness Central, 2003. See also Dr. Young's website.

Clinical Oncology for Medical Students and Physicians, op. cit, pp.32, 34

Spontaneous Regression of Cancer: "The Metabolic Triumph of the Host!", op. cit.,pp. 136, 137.

Manner, HW, Michaelson, TL, and DiSanti, SJ. "Enzymatic Analysis of Normal and Malignant Tissues." Presented at the Illinois State Academy of Science, April 1978. Also, Manner, HW, Michaelson, TL, and DiSanti, SJ, "Amygdalin, Vitamin A and Enzymes Induced Regression of Murine Mammary Adenocarcinomas", Journal of Manipulative and Physiological Therapeutics, Vol 1, No. 4, December 1978. 200 East Roosevelt Road, Lombard, IL 60148 USA

Vitamin B15 (Pangamic Acid); Properties, Functions, and Use. (Moscow: Science Publishing House, 1965), translated and reprinted by McNaughton Foundation, Sausalito, Calif.

Catalona, et al. Medical World News, 6/23/72, pg 82M California cancer Advisory council, 1963, pg 10 Weilerstein, R. W., ACS Volunteer, 19, #1, 1973

Burger, Hospital Practice, July, 1973, 55-62

Currie & Bagshawe, Lancet, 1, (7492), 708, 1967

Abercrombie, Ca. Res. 22, 525, 1962

Cormack, Ca. Res. 30, (5), 1459, 1970

Catalona, et al. Medical World News, 6/23/72, pg 82M

Jose, Nut. Today, March, 1973, pgs 4-9

Burk & Winzler, VITAMINS AND HORMONES, vol. II, 1944

Adcock et al, Science, 181, 8/31/73, 845-47

Dr. Dean Burk formerly chief of cytochemistry, The National cancer institute, and Dr. John Yiamouyiannis, Science Director of The National Health Federation, Formerly an editor of chemical Abstracts.

Fairley, Brit. Med. J. 2,1969, 467-473

Burk, McNaughton, Von Ardenne, PanMinerva Med. 13, #12, Dec. 1971

Lea, et al, ca. Res. 35, 2321 -2326, Sept. 1975

The McNaughton Foundation, I.N.D. 6734, April 6, 1970

Nieper, Krebsgeschehen, 4,1972

J.A.M.A. 225, 4, July, 1973, pg 424

Shamberger et al, Proc. Nat, Acad. Sci. May, 1973

Shute & Shute, ALPHA TOCOPHEROL IN CARDIOVASCULAR DISEASE, Ryerson Press, Toronto, Canada, 1954

Ransberger, 10th Int. Cancer Congress, 1970

Wolf & Ransberger, ENZYME THERAPY, Vantage Pr. 1972

Summa; Dipl. Ing. (Chem) Landstuhl, 1972

Reitnauer, Arzneim. Forsch. 22, 1347-61, 1972

Folkman, Ann. Surg. 175, (3). 409-1 6, 1972

Penn, 7th Annual Cancer Conf. 1973

The MEDICAL LETTER, vol. 15, #3 (issue #367) 2/2/73

Kreuger, ADVANCES IN PHARM. & CHEMOTHERAPY, vol x, 1973

Annals New York Academy of Science: 164, 2, 1969

Sorbo, Acta Chem. Scand. 5, 1951, (724-34); 1953 (1129-1136); 1953 (1137-1145)

Clemedson et al, Acta Physiol. Scand. 32, 1954, 245

Engel, Med. Klink. 20, 1790, 1930

DeFermo, Arch. Ital. de Chir. 33: 801, 1933

Saphir,~Endocrinol. 18, 191, 1934

Velasquez & Engel, Endocrinol. 27, 523, 1940

Li, Med. Clin N. Am. 45, 661 -666, May, 1961

Roffo, Bol. Inst. de Med. 21, 41 9-586, 1944

Friedman, Ann. N.Y. Acad. Sci. 80-1 61, 1959 (and refs)

Krebs & Gurchot, Science, 104, 302, 1946

Braunstein, et al, Annals Int. Med. 78:39-45, 1973

Naughton et al, Ca. Res. 35, 1887-1 890, July, 1975

Wide & Gemzell, Acta Endocrinol. 35-261, 1960

Navarro, 9th International Cancer Congress, Toyko, Oct. 1966 reported in HEALTH AND LIGHT, by John Ott, D.Sc., Devin Adair, 1973

Nieper, Agressologie 12, 6,1971, 401-8

Livingston, CANCER: A NEW BREAKTHROUGH, Nash Publishing, Los Angeles, 1972

Benno C. Schmidt, chairman of the Memorial Sloan-Kettering Cancer Center, New York City, chairman of The President's Cancer Panel; address to the A.C.S., California

Division, Oct. 12, 1973 (Los Angeles Times)
Yudkin, SWEET AND DANGEROUS, Bantam Books, 1972
Seminars on Healing, The Academy of Parapsychology and Medicine, June 1973

Torrance & Schnabel, Ann. Intern. Med. 6, 732, 1932
Leivy & Schnabel, Am. I. Med. Sd. 183, 381, 1932
Gillette, et al, I. Clin. Invest. 51, 36a, 1972
Gillette, et al, New Eng. J. Med. 290, 654, 1974
Cerami & Manning, Prac. Natl. Acad. Sci. 68, 1180, 1971
Gillette et al, ibid, 68, 2791, 1971
Cerami, et al, Fed. Proc. 32, 1668, 1973
Manning, et al, Adv. Exp. Med. Biol. 28, 253, 1972
Houston, Am. Laboratory, 7, #10, October, 1975 (and editorial)
DeLange & Ermans, Am. I. Clin. Nut. 24, 1354, 1971
Barnes, Broda, M.D., HEART ATTACK RARENESS IN THYROID-TREATED PA
TIENTS, C.C. Thomas, 1972
Barnes and Galton, HYPOTHYROIDISM, THE UNSUSPECTED ILLNESS, Thomas Y.
Crowell, N.Y., Feb. 1976
Smith, J. C. Medical Counterpoint, Nov. 1973
Oberleas, Intntl. Trace Elements Symp. Modern Med., Sept. 16, 1974
New Scientist, 5/2/74
Korant, B.D., Nature, 4/12/74
Klenner, FR., I. So. Med. & Surg. 111, 209, 1949
Stacpoole, P.W., Med. Hyp., March-April, 1975
C.A. Dombradi and S. Foldeak, "Screening Report on the Antitumor Activity of Purified
Arctium Lappa Extracts," Tumori, vol. 52, 1966, p. 173, cited in Patricia Spain Ward,
"History of Hoxsey Treatment," contract report for the U.S. Congress, Office of
Technology Assessment, May 1988.
Kazuyoshi Morita, Tsuneo Kada, and Mitsuo Namiki, "A Desmutagenic Factor Isolated
From Burdock (Arctium Lappa Linne)," Mutation Research, vol. 129, 1984, pp. 25-31,
cited in Patricia Spain Ward, "History of Hoxsey Treatment," contract report for the U.S.
Congress, Office of Technology Assessment, May 1988.

Sheila Snow Fraser and Carroll Allen, "Could Essiac Halt Cancer?" Homemaker's, June-
July August 1977, p. 19.
"Essiac as an Aid in Surgery," Bracebridge Examiner, 13 March 1991.
Gary L. Glum, Calling of an Angel (Los Angeles: Silent Walker Publishing, 1988), p.
i."Essiac Added 18 Years to Her Mother's Life," Bracebridge Examiner, 6 February
1991.7. "Cancer Commission Was Nothing But a Farce," Bracebridge Examiner, 9
January 1991.8. Glum, op. cit., p. 136.9. Ibid.

S. J. Haught. Censured for Curing Cancer: The American Experience of Dr. Max Gerson.
San Diego: The Gerson Institute, 1991.
Tanya Harter Pierce M.A., MFCC, "Outsmart your cancer" 2004.

Richard Walters. *Options: The Alternative Cancer Therapy Book*. New York: Avery Penguin Putnam, 1993.
James P. Carter, M.D. *Racketeering in Medicine: The Suppression of Alter- natives*. Hampton Roads, 1993.
Ross Pelton and Lee Overholser. *Alternatives in Cancer Therapy*. New York: Simon and Schuster, 1994.

DISCARD

31188965R00106

MAY -- 2016

3475662

Made in the USA
Middletown, DE
21 April 2016